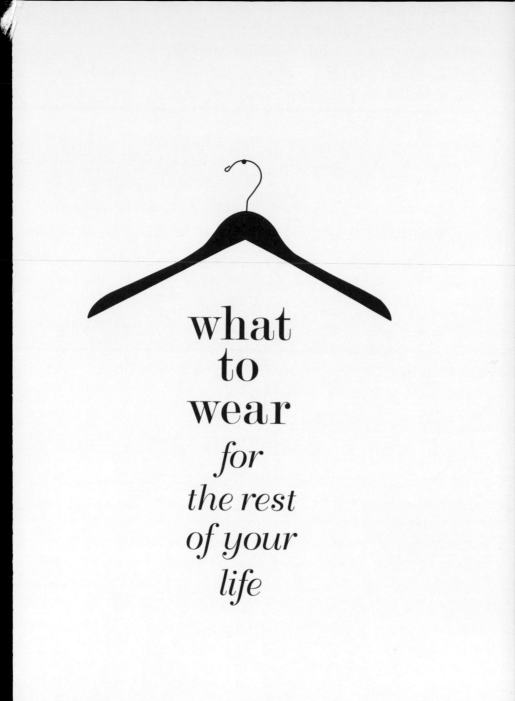

what
to
wear
for
the rest
of your
life

what to wear

for the rest of your

wear

to

life

AGELESS SECRETS OF STYLE

Kim Johnson Gross

SPRINGBOARD

New York • Boston

Springboard Press
Hachette Book Group
237 Park Avenue, New York, NY 10017

www.HachetteBookGroup.com

Springboard Press is an imprint of Grand Central Publishing. The Springboard Press
name and logo are trademarks of Hachette Book Group, Inc.

Printed in Singapore

First Edition: May 2010
10 9 8 7 6 5 4 3 2 1

Library of Congress Cataloging-in-Publication Data
Gross, Kim Johnson.
What to wear for the rest of your life: ageless secrets of style / Kim Johnson Gross.—
1st ed.
    p. cm.
ISBN 978-0-446-53494-9
1. Fashion. 2. Women's clothing. 3. Beauty, Personal. 4. Aging. I. Title.
TT507.G735 2010
646.7'042–dc22
2009015447

Design by Wayne Wolf/Blue Cup Creative

For my precious daughters Glenna and Carolyn who inspired me,
each in her own way, to share my story.
For my Style and Life Mentor, my mother Evelyn Johnson.
For my dad, Glenn Johnson, who is keeping watch.
For Jeff who makes me laugh every day.

With love and gratitude.

We are not human beings
on a spiritual journey.
We are spiritual beings
on a human journey.

—Stephen Covey

Why see a shrink?
You'll feel much better
if you spend the money
on a new dress.

—Evelyn Johnson, my mother

Contents

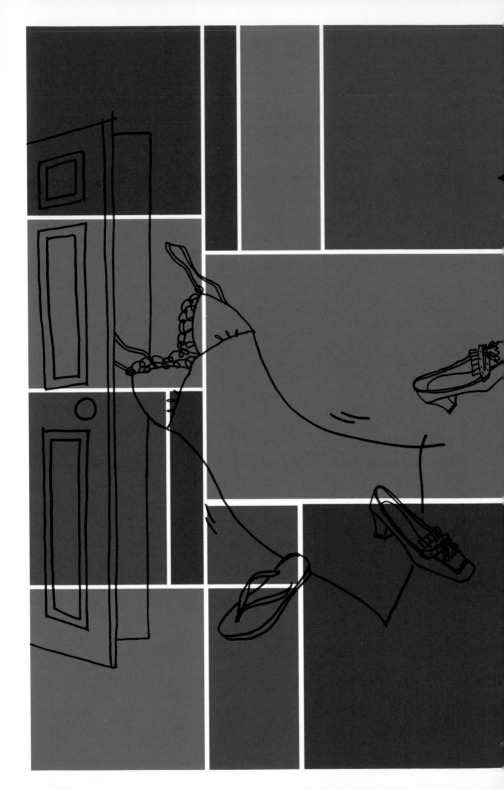

> How many cares one loses when one decides not to be something, but someone.
>
> —Coco Chanel

PART ONE
HOW SHOULD I LOOK?

> Middle-aged women have a lot in common with kids—all of us are on the cusp of the unknown: enticing and scary.
>
> —Jane Pauley, *Skywriting: A Life Out of the Blue*

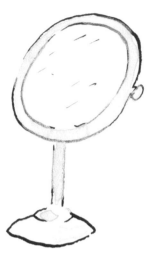

1

Endings and Beginnings

I woke up one morning and couldn't believe this was my life. I had turned fifty, sent my youngest daughter to college, closed my business, divorced, and none of my clothes fit. Not only had my life changed, but my body was changing, without my permission! I could no longer count on my clothes to get me through any occasion, special or not. They seemed to have shrunk overnight. I'd look in the mirror and wonder *How do I look?*—and suspect it wasn't the way I had long imagined. Was it really the way I appeared in photographs—the fuller face, weaker chin, and thicker middle, much like my dad? Was I growing into my genes while growing out of my jeans? I was confused, but my mother wasn't.

I didn't want to believe it—my ever-supportive mother disapproving of me? Her sunny demeanor froze as she looked me up and down while I was wearing the bikini my sister Jill had given me for my fiftieth birthday. I'd like to think it was a gift my sister thought I'd look good wearing, rather than a challenge or taunt. At forty-seven, Jill remained trim, while my body had gradually betrayed my genetics, most notably my dad's flabby stomach.

But my mother's stinging assessment shocked me: "*You must lose weight and never wear a two-piece again!*" Granted she is a stylish and fit octogenarian, but I'm no slouch. And although I have built a successful career as a style expert, I really couldn't see why she was so upset. Her rebuke reminded me of an afternoon when I was nineteen, lounging around my friend Bella's pool, sneaking surreptitious glances at her uncle's new wife wearing a tiny bikini. Aunt Katje had a tanned leathered face and pillowy flesh swelled around her middle, making her look old and careless to me. Looking back, I suspect she was only in her forties. I was simultaneously repulsed and intrigued. Was that what my mother was feeling now?

Aunt Katje lived in France and Sweden with Bella's uncle, an architect. They were creative intellectuals who traveled the world. He designed buildings; she wrote about art and food. There was something strangely glamorous about Aunt Katje—was it the substantial gold hoop earrings she wore, along with the kicky mules and colorful sarong that she unwrapped to tan her practically naked body? Or that she seemed utterly comfortable in her skin? Acutely aware that I wasn't, I suspected that her allure had much to do with her self-confidence.

In the years since, I have acquired my own wrinkles and fleshy middle. I have also gained a certain amount of wisdom and confidence, and needed all of it that day to cope with my mother's piercing words. A mother's opinion has an impact. I longed for her guidance, not her consternation. It took writing this story, which first appeared in *More Magazine*, for me to understand that her reaction was primal: a mother wanting her divorced daughter to attract, remarry, be loved and taken care of by a man. Only then could she rest in peace. I have similar dreams, but if I were to constantly try to recapture a youthful appearance to "get" the man and not enjoy who I am at any age, what kind of relationship would that be between him and me—and worse, between me and myself? One of high anxiety, I suspect.

Little did I know then that this incident was to be the start of many more closet challenges. I was entering a new phase in my life and was determined to make the very best of it. I had to rethink the way I had been dressing for the last thirty years. It was time for a fresh start.

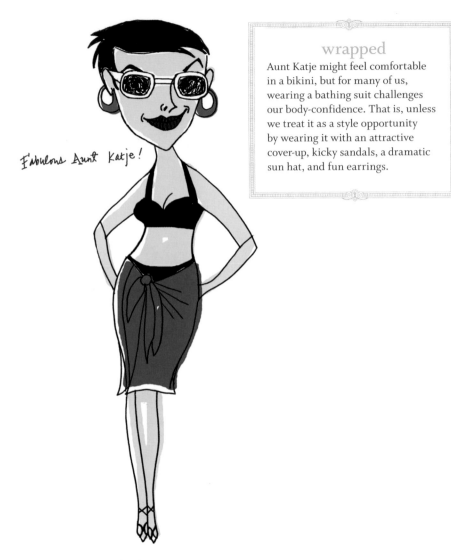

Fabulous Aunt Katje!

Aunt Katje's Secret

Aunt Katje is European. Even in adolescence, my unworldly eyes suspected that was the mystery of her allure.

European women and men honor their lifetime of experiences and their physical manifestations. They enjoy the sensuality of everyday life, whether it's sex, a ripe peach, or the feel of cashmere against their bodies. They respect the powerful connection between what they wear and how they feel. We, too, can adapt aspects of their approach to life to gain our own clothes-body-life-confidence.

DRESS FOR YOUR OWN PLEASURE.

TAKE CARE OF YOUR SKIN. A Paris-based research company polled three hundred European women and asked what they would take with them to Mars. The number one choice was moisturizer, ahead of husbands.

HAVE AN AWARENESS AND APPRECIATION OF THE EVERYDAY CHOICES YOU MAKE. The tea you choose to drink and the cup you drink it from; the sheets and pillow you nestle into at night; how you want to feel in the clothes you wear.

SENSUALIZE YOUR SENSES.
   Touch. Wear fabrics that feel good against your skin. Cotton is as desirable as cashmere depending on thread count. The higher it is, the more luxurious it feels.
   Sound. The click of heels, the romance of jazz, the jangle of bracelets, the joy of a laugh (laugh lines are sexier than no lines).
   Taste. A kiss, the taste of ripe fruit—take time to enjoy.
   Scent. Freshly picked herbs, a breeze of salt water, the body of someone you love. Pheromones are a scent secreted to attract the opposite sex.
   Sight. If it is aesthetically pleasing to your eye, enjoy. If not, keep experimenting.

WISDOM IS SEXY. Flirting is sexy. Lingerie is sexy. Sex is sexy. Mature women are sexy.

BEAUTY HAS NO EXPIRATION DATE.

STYLE DOESN'T AGE, IT EVOLVES.

2

Closet Betrayal

My closet ditched me for a younger woman. I should have seen it coming long before staking out a pharmacy in a town where I would not likely run into someone I knew. Buying an over-the-counter pregnancy kit requires discretion. Ha! It had been close to twenty years since I'd felt this particular kind of anticipation, yet I was perversely giddy that the girl in me might still have what it takes, and a pregnancy would surely explain my burgeoning stomach.

My inner voice—the sane one—mocked me knowingly. I had as much chance of being pregnant as I had of navigating a map without reading glasses and massive amounts of light. But I wouldn't allow myself any other explanation for the swelling in the middle of my body that had ballooned over the last few months, alienating me from myself along with everything in my closet.

Granted, my closet and I have had our ups and our downs over the last few years, but we had muddled our way through them. I started keeping a few sizes of pants on hand for some of my good-weight weeks and some for my not-so-good ones. And retiring the fashionista wardrobe that dominated my closet for the twenty-nine years I worked in New York City had caught us both off-guard. I had decided to sell my business and shift gears to write full-time. I loved the idea of no longer going to an office—even better, not being responsible for one—and relished the freedom to work anywhere in the world that had broadband access.

The reality: Two years after having the good fortune of doing what I wished for, I was spending too much time at home alone working at my computer, which is not only psychically challenging but also physically tough on the back and waistline. As a style expert, you might expect that I would have dressed for my day in the "office," even though it was only arm's length from my refrigerator. To be brutally honest, there were soon plenty of days when there was no distinguishing the clothes I slept in from those I worked in, unless I ventured out to a yoga class or dinner with a friend. I let myself drift into that mistake. As our lives change, our closets often bear the brunt.

Closet Confidential: *Moving On*

"The transition was hard on my closet when I left the corporate world. For ten years, I had worn serious suits. They were very nice and expensive and I didn't want to let them go, but I no longer liked how I felt wearing them. They were the clothes of a different person. One who managed people, reported to the president (of a prestigious beauty company), conducted meetings and presentations, and was responsible for sales projections. The new me wanted to let the creative out. Until recently, my closet was still transitioning out some of those corporate suits. It's been eight years, and I've finally let them go."

Susan, fifty-two, design entrepreneur, Manhattan

Closets are powerful. They contain the power to make us feel fat, fit, frumpy, or fabulous. Yet each of us holds the power to shape our closets and the way we want them to make us feel. If disciplined, we can refigure them each season to adapt to our changing needs. Emotionally, they measure the seasons of our lives. Closets house our memories, dreams, fantasies, aspirations, inspirations, expectations, relationships, mistakes, triumphs, frustrations, adventures, joys, and failures—our stories. Closets hold our autobiographies, and with mindfulness, what we choose to share them with can help us decide how we want to continue to write our own story.

Transitions make for especially crowded closets. The uncertainty we experience makes it difficult to decide what to hang on to and what to let go of. The clothes that had once defined us may no longer fit with who we are now. In the past, career suits might have replaced mini skirts, but what replaces those suits now? Our thrill for prom dresses faded long before we shopped for a wedding dress. A maternity wardrobe was an easy fix for a changing body. After we perfunctorily ditched it, we wondered what to hang in its place—the body had changed, as had the identity. Now we are dressing to be the mother of the bride or maybe perhaps the encore bride. As our self-image is once again challenged, we look within our closet to salvage what we can.

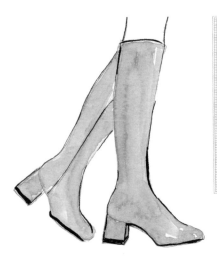

to boot

In the mid-sixties, designer André Courrèges introduced go-go boots in white plastic. They were the rage, and complemented the mini, also a favorite of the times. Ever since, low-heeled mid-calf, knee-high, and over-the-knee boots have been Closet Classics.

When I was sixteen, I worked weekends in the local Pappagallo shop, where for the first time ever I made enough money to shape my closet the way I wanted to. It was the late 1960s and Diana Vreeland was editor in chief of *Vogue*. She transformed the elegant, lady-like magazine my mother had subscribed to into one that was visually modern, exotic, daring, sensual, and packed with energy. Her pages opened my eyes to a new way of looking at clothes, at beauty, and at a world bigger than the one I knew. I taped over the rose chintz wallpaper that covered my bedroom walls with pages I had ripped from the magazine—Avedon's portraits of the lanky English model Twiggy with her cropped hair and exaggerated false eyelashes wearing mod clothes hot from Carnaby Street boutiques and flower power face paint. Her stick figure and petite breasts helped me feel more comfortable with my own similar build. There were portraits of

Masai warriors in native dress photographed on white seamless paper in a photographer's studio rather than their natural turf, and mesmerizing pages of models wearing dramatic clothes in cinematic locations—palaces, mosques, remote villages in countries I knew little about. I wanted to travel the world these pages captured.

Vreeland's *Vogue* re-created the norm of "beauty," favoring models of pedigree whose looks were intriguing—Penelope Tree was described by the famed English photographer David Bailey as an "Elfin Jiminy Cricket"; "Queen of the Scene" Marisa Berenson's glamour gave confidence to girls with curly hair and not-so-perfect noses, while Veruschka's imposing six-foot-plus, often body-painted physique emboldened a generation of young women to feel better about their bodies, whatever their height.

In the 1960s, Pappagallo's ultra-feminine flat tassel loafer was a winning mix of buttery leather and happy color combinations—yellow and blue, green and pink, blue and green. They, along with Jack Rogers's Navajo sandals and Belgian shoes, were the casual shoe of choice in WASP playgrounds such as Palm Beach, Newport, Lyford Cay, and Locust Valley, where I grew up.

Kate Spade wore them in high school. Wendy Wasserstein immortalized their cult pedigree in *Shiksa Goddess*, a collection of essays:

> I was speaking at the Lion of Judah luncheon in Palm Beach recently when I noticed a woman in a Lilly Pulitzer dress, one strand of pearls, and forty-year-old pink Pappagallo shoes leaning against the door. She stood out from the crowd because, instead of the omnipresent Barry Kieselstein-Cord purse with lizard clasp, she was carrying a battered lacrosse stick.

Forty-year-old Pappagallos! I wish I had hung on to mine. I can't even find them on eBay. I may have better luck finding a pair in my mother's closet.

Couture was no longer the standard-bearer of fashion. *Vogue* featured the clothes of change, inspired by our generation's street wear. Their cadre of supermodels leaped across the pages showing us how to wear our mini skirts in a better way—in crisply cut styles patterned in bold colorful graphics accessorized with huge faux jewelry, patent go-go boots, and wildly configured hair extensions that were intended to appear artificially decorative, rather than a subtle embellishment.

These pages inspired me to look at clothes differently. They could have personality and pizzazz, break the rules. Besides all that, they looked fun to wear. I filled my closet with more affordable but no less dynamic versions of the featured paper dresses, gladiator sandals, faux hair extensions, and overblown papier-mâché jewelry. When I wasn't rolling up the waistline of my skirts after school, I wore minis in op art patterns and neon colors that glowed as brilliantly under the ultraviolet lights of Cheetah, The Electric Circus, Le Club, and other New York City discotheques, as they did in the rec rooms in our parents' basements that my friends and I more likely frequented.

Before, my closet had been under my mother's watch, but now it was my sanctuary—a place where I could experiment with fashion that reflected the prevailing culture at any given moment. Essentially I learned to weed out old trends to make room for the new. This process, which I now refer to as "Assess, Dejunk, and Renew," was the way I learned to define and refine my style.

> The Chic Simple book series that I created with Jeff Stone in the 1990s comprised guides to simplifying life with economy and style. Part of the process was to Assess, Dejunk, and Renew the various closets in our lives—clothes, kitchen, bedroom, beauty—seasonally to keep us, and our closets, in sync with changes in our bodies, our lives, and our style.

Unlike my mother the pack rat, I recycled things in my closet that I no longer fancied or that didn't fit my body or my life. Sure, I wish I had kept some of my 1960s regalia, but the mod go-go boots I wore to a Beatles concert at Shea Stadium in 1967 would have looked ridiculous as I trudged through the mud two years later amid the tie-dyed and jeans revolutionary culture at Woodstock. Besides, I am not one to lug around remnants of my life. I was always looking forward, not backward. Now I'm not quite sure what I'm looking forward to.

3

Assess, Dejunk, and Renew

Assess, Dejunk, and Renew is a seasonal practice to keep you and your closet in sync with the changes in your body, your life, and your style.

Step 1: Assess

EXAMINE YOUR LIFE and think about what you need to wear for it. The career wardrobe I cultivated for twenty-plus years doesn't fit my body or my life now. Since I've started writing from home, my daily uniform has shifted from suits, of which I had many, to sport and casual clothes, which were once negligible.

CHECK YOUR CALENDAR. Do you have any special upcoming events that require special attention to what you want to wear? When you match your clothes with your life, it will give your closet focus.

Step 2: Dejunk

This step is a reality check. It requires time, patience, honesty, a full-length mirror, and good lighting. Try on your clothes each season to check for fit (it's likely your weight has shifted in the last year), then decide what you continue to enjoy wearing, what needs to be tailored, and what still suits your life. If you don't have the time this requires, start with one category of clothing at a time.

RECYCLE those things that no longer work, otherwise they'll crowd your closet and your mind. It takes courage to let go of those clothes from a life and body that were. I enjoy not wearing a suit for every workday anymore, but I'm annoyed when my jeans no longer fit. Rather than keeping a closet filled with clothes that make me feel bad about myself, I sell or give the offenders away, which makes the sting less painful.

Despite how disciplined I am, there inevitably are items I continue to hang on to. A favorite black cocktail dress sits quietly waiting to come out of retirement (it's those five-plus pounds I promise to lose). I've kept a favorite micro-mini skirt for decades in hope that one of my daughters might eventually enjoy wearing it as much as I did. Maybe this season I'll get real and convert it into a pillow. But mostly I hang on to these items and a few others because they have been woven with memories, much like Proust's madeleine.

> In Marcel Proust's master work *Remembrance of Things Past,* the taste of a madeleine (a cake-like cookie in a scalloped shape similar to a seashell) transports the narrator from feeling captive by the mundane bleakness of his everyday life into a beguiling world of memory.

What we keep is as telling as what we choose not to. It's part of the magic closets hold.

Closet Confidential: Memory Closets

Cynthia, a bicoastal gal whose enthralling life stories read like an Edith Wharton novel, keeps a closet filled with the fabulous clothes she wore as a young woman to remind her of the glamorous life she led. She even dated Cary Grant!

Diane is a worldly sixty-four-year-old New Yorker who considers a number of her clothes her friends. A great many hold treasured remembrances of the exciting life she shared with her late husband. She values their company even if they sometimes no longer fit her or her currently quieter life.

> Sally had a closet stuffed with clothes until a friend gave her a gift of a "closet specialist" to help sort things out. They dejunked maternity clothes and the broad-shouldered business suits that were stylish in the 1980s, when she was a music attorney. But there were other things she wanted to hang on to knowing she would never wear them again. They held an emotional connection she was not prepared to give up. She archived them in long canvas bags that now hang in her cedar attic.

DEJUNKING is also when you get to shop your closet. Because we wear 20 percent of our clothes 80 percent of the time, we tend to lose track of what we own, especially if our closets are overstuffed.

The last time I cleaned out my closet, I found clothes with the price tags on.
—Lise, fifty-four, attorney, Providence, Rhode Island

By getting into your closet each season, you are likely to unearth some treasures or give new life to clothes you already own by wearing them in new ways. If velvet is the rave, mix your velvet pieces with your other basics for a fresh look. The pants of your favorite suit may no longer fit, but pairing the jacket with jeans will make each look modern.

Step 3: Renew

What's left? Do you have what you need? Do you like what you have? If not, start a Shop Smart list to keep track of those things you need before you shop. Shopping with focus will help keep you within your budget and make your closet a happy one.

Assess, Dejunk, and Renew is a practice I apply when evaluating other aspects of my life—career, friends, where to live. As my goals and life change, I am constantly assessing what matters to me, and jettisoning what doesn't.

Caring Closet

The Container Store's website is a great source of closet solutions. The folks there advise that the best way to protect your clothes against moths, dust, fading, and mildew is to "Clean, Contain, and Repel." I have lost some of my favorite dresses, sweaters, and gloves by not heeding this advice.

Clean. Moths and carpet beetles are closet enemy number one. They wreak havoc on natural fibers and chow down on food stains within synthetic fibers. So before you store your clothes, clean them, even if you don't think you have a problem. Once a moth lays its eggs, your clothes will age to look like a fine Swiss cheese. To be safe, store clothes off-season with a sachet or canister containing repellents. Those containing paradichlorobenzene will not permeate clothes with the lingering scent of naphthalene found in old-fashioned mothballs. If you already have a problem, most clothes can be sprayed with an insecticide spray also containing paradichlorobenzene, which kills pests on contact.

Contain. Protective storage containers come in a variety of shapes, sizes, and materials. Unbleached cotton is best for storing natural fibers including leathers and fur because it allows them to breathe.

Sturdy vinyl storage bags offer visibility.

Clear storage boxes with locking lids, and with the option of wheels, are like portable drawers.

Repel. All-natural cedar is fragrant to people and their pets—unless of course you're into breeding moths and carpet beetles, which are repelled by the scent. Lavender, rosemary, eucalyptus, mint, and thyme are just a few of the herbs often mixed into sachets that are natural deterrents to those pesky pests.

Line storage bags with cedar for extra protection.

4

Déjà Vu: Here We Go Again

My closet had always been in evolution. Now I was trying to cope with revolution. Unlike the other physical changes that had gradually nestled into my closet without much fanfare—an increasingly abundant supply of reading glasses to accommodate not only failing eyes but also another new change, forgetting where I've left them; the upswing of flats and other nurturing shoes, because I had long since convinced myself that comfort is its very own chic; an assortment of body-shaping underwear for when I chose to wear undies at all; pull-on pants with elastic waistbands (don't cringe, they actually can look and feel good if the waistband lies flat and there are seams that provide curves)—this change in my closet was different. This lump on my stomach landed like an alien from nowhere, without warning and without apparent logic. Whatever the reason, it posed a challenge to my closet and my psyche that could not be ignored. This was no longer a quick Spanx fix. It was an outer-body experience, not dissimilar to witnessing my body unfold without control during puberty.

> Spanx was founded by Sara Blakely in 1998 when she cut the feet off a pair of pantyhose to wear under white pants and open-toed shoes. In 2000, the footless pantyhose made Oprah's Favorite Things list. Their motto *No more grid butt!* is apt for their expansive line of body shapers, including control fishnets.

While our memories may not be terrific anymore, most of us remember the angst of adolescence. Our bodies were developing as our hormones raged. The crucial what-to-wear questions were bra or no bra (when-ohwhen in my case) and how padded if we dared. Even if our chests didn't need a boost, our confidence did.

When I was fifteen, my mother was even more panicked than me that my breasts were not noticeably filling out. Now she's panicked that I am filling out everything all too well. I was locked in the self-conscious adolescent horror of not knowing how, when, or even if my body was really going to unfold into womanhood. My mother encouraged me to wear padded bras. I literally dipped my toe into these new waters when I wore a formfitting bathing suit with ample bra cups on a seriously hormonal beach during a spring break in Fort Lauderdale. I felt as though I were trying on a body that I quite liked, but didn't own. When I emerged from the ocean after a swim, I was startled by a loud slurping noise. The bra cups had inverted. I looked like Madonna from a different universe. The horror of being found out rocked my pubescent mind.

Once again raging hormones are hijacking my body in ways I can't seem to control. I feel as though I am undergoing a second puberty filled with the same insecurity of the unknown, and it's wreaking havoc on my closet.

The over-the-counter pregnancy test I took was negative. A swollen or bloated stomach is also one of the many symptoms of ovarian cancer, so I had a pelvic examination and a vaginal sonogram, which can help to detect a tumor. My thyroid was also tested, because scant menstruation, weight gain, and dry skin can be signs of trouble. The good news:

Closet Confidential: *Now and Then*

"I always thought my looks were a birthright, not something I had to work for. I was a good student, pretty, had a personality everyone liked and a tight little body, all of which I took for granted. I didn't notice when it ended. I got thicker in the middle when I was thirty-five. Then after a partial hysterectomy I gained fifteen pounds, which gradually increased to another nine. I might have been upset, but I had great professional things happening that distracted me. Then the business was sold and the entire staff was let go. I was upset and didn't care about my appearance. Before, I had an image in my head of how I'd look when I was mature, and I enjoyed that image. Suddenly I realized I didn't look like 'her.'"

Marilyn, sixty-plus, Internet entrepreneur, Chatham, New York

All tests were negative. The news: My doctor confirmed I was in menopause.

How am I supposed to look? Who am I dressing for anyway? Should I worry about others' expectations? And who exactly do I consider "others," and what do I imagine are their expectations? What can I control and what can't I? Should I get a little nip and tuck to remove the Alien growing on my middle, and a few other things while I'm at it?

I'd like to think that I didn't care about the superficiality of it all, but I had lost my inner bearing, because of my outer changes. Until now, I hadn't realized how much my appearance or my closet had defined me personally and professionally—as a young Ford model wearing fashion, as an advertising designer selling the allure of fashion, as a magazine editor and columnist covering fashion, and as creator of a style brand and books.

The closets we keep mirror our "reality"—who we were, who we are, and who we want to be. Every time we dress or buy something to wear, we are making a choice. It is a tangible affirmation of how we define ourselves, which can be confusing when we're in the throes of redefining our self-image and re-dressing our new and unfamiliar body. When we dress to feel our best, we nurture the woman we are and strive to be.

> ### Closet Confidential: *Fashion Breakdown*
> "I had always used fashion as an expression of my inner feelings, but when I turned forty-three, I had a fashion breakdown. I needed to come to terms with my age and stage in life in terms of my closet."
>
> *Peggy, forty-four, Realtor, Los Angeles*

As a fashion expert, I knew that what I wore was the one thing I could control when everything else seemed out of control. My current closet chaos signaled that I was entering a new phase in my life—and I was determined to make the very best of it. I had to rethink the way I had been dressing for the last thirty years. It was time for a fresh start.

5

The Lying Mirror

I had wanted to believe that my body would remain young forever. The infallible self-image that I had held for so long was of an attractive, youthful, strong, energetic woman who would always be the tall, slim one in a crowd. Then the visual in my mind's eye that I had long negotiated with the mirror completely shattered when an elegant older woman in tai chi class commented on how gracefully I moved considering I was pregnant. I knew that the mirror had been lying, but my clothes weren't. Clearly I was not dressing my best. The closet that had been a safe haven was elevated to code red.

For the next several months, I avoided my closet, the mirror, my mother, women I hadn't seen in a while, and my ex-husband—I didn't want to give him or his girlfriend the satisfaction of seeing that I didn't look like the youthful girl I had long imagined.

In *Why Beauty Matters*, a paper published in the March 2006 *American Economic Review*, economists Markus M. Mobius of Harvard and Tanya S. Rosenblat of Wesleyan reported on an experiment they conducted to determine if beauty was a premium in the workplace. Students were recruited to role-play employers and job applicants interviewing for a job involving mazes. The results? Appearance had no impact on productivity, but beautiful people were more confident in their abilities, which employers interpreted as a sign of increased productivity. This helped explain why beautiful men and women are the first to get hired and are often paid more than their colleagues.

Seeing colleagues in fashion felt especially threatening. I now lacked the confidence for their scrutiny. Far too many have remained preternaturally thin, and without the wrinkles or droopiness that belies age. Any slip is considered a lack of discipline—and worse, a sign of aging, which in a field of "outer" can be considered a career detriment. At least that's what I felt now being on the flip side of the equation. I was actually told by an editor before the Alien landed on my stomach that she was upset because the very accomplished actress who was about to appear on the cover of the magazine she edited looked fat. Granted, she looked not like an anorexic, cinematic pinup girl, but like an acknowledged talent and beauty with much wisdom to share. No wonder many of us experience confusion when our inner selves are challenged by the outer standards that permeate our lives. What's chilling is that the number of women over forty suffering from eating disorders is rapidly growing.

According to a report on MSNBC, a study from the Eating Disorder Center of Denver has confirmed that an increasing number of women in midlife (thirty-five to sixty-five) are struggling with dangerous and potentially deadly eating disorders. The author of the study, Dr. Tamara Pryor, refers to this phenomenon as the "Desperate Housewives" effect, because of how slim and young the middle-aged women on the popular television show appear. She puts some responsibility on the culture that supports and encourages "fountain of youth fixes" whereby many older women feel pressured to appear young and slender even though it's not normal for women over thirty to have the same bodies they did at eighteen.

Closet Confidential: *Picture Perfect*

Anne remains a captive of the photographs she surrounds herself with. They document her incredible beauty when she was a young star in New York City intelligentsia. She remains innately chic and enormously talented, but she can't reconcile herself to the body she dwells in forty years after the photographs were taken. She holds herself hostage to a memory that remains alive only in her mind's eye by choosing to hide from life as best she can, waiting. Waiting for what? I consider her a magnificent talent—even admiring the way she dresses up the body she loathes.

Anne's withdrawal is a cautionary tale. Nothing can bring back physical youth. Time only honors the present. When we attempt to deny our age, we become more fearful of it. Only when we accept ourselves at this very moment can we experience the joy of not being eternally nagged by the "what-if" or the "wait-until," or mourn the "what-was," and get on with our lives. And by dressing our body best, we honor the body we have now.

I got focused. I decided to own up to my new body, rather than continue to hide in dread or, worse, give up on me. I needed to accept my body in the present rather than try in vain to recapture the body that was. I began to recognize the importance of being a role model to my daughters—hell, I needed to be a role model to myself! If I could experience menopause and live the next part of my life with grace, vitality, personal growth, and style, then this could be a gift of sorts for them and for me.

> As women, we're lucky because we are reminded in a very physical way that this is midlife, so we can reevaluate what we are and where we're going . . . It's very healthy to view menopause as a chance to recharge and rebuild.
> —Dr. Susan Love, surgeon, quoted in *Fifty on Fifty* by Bonnie Miller Rubin

I began telling everyone that the Alien was my menopause. I was declaring to the world, and more importantly to myself, that I was entering a new and natural time of my life. My daughters were embarrassed by my candor, which meant they were paying attention, and I was starting to Assess, Dejunk, and Renew my self-image. I needed to become reacquainted with my body before dealing with my closet.

6

Closet Health

What was this new body of mine about? This transition was not just about my closet, which clearly freaked me out as a fashion professional, but also about my health. I had my fears. If the Alien could invade without warning, what other surprises might be lurking within?

One of my younger sisters had already successfully battled breast cancer shortly after turning fifty, and my mother had done so twice after menopause. I am built like my father—long, lean limbs centered by weight, mostly stored in the stomach. Golf was his sport until his feet became infected from the effects of Type 2 diabetes, exacerbated by his sugar addiction. He became depressed. My parents thought psychiatric treatment a sign of weakness and a waste of money. He preferred to retreat into the cloud of cigarette smoke he had long found comfort in. He died when he was sixty-six from heart disease. My father was reckless with his physical and mental health. I did not want the same fate.

Other tests I had undergone to help determine the cause of the Alien revealed that my blood pressure was good and my cholesterol levels were terrible. And obviously to the eye, my metabolism had slowed to what appeared to be a screeching halt. My well-respected male doctors told me menopause didn't warrant weight gain. They advised me to lose three and a half pounds a month until I'd shed the fifteen-pound Alien. The more I tried, the more I gained. I felt like a loser.

These doctors sounded like an ex (or so I imagined) and the fashion crowd I was hiding from. Thankfully a female doctor explained what was going on. As women's hormones change with age, our bodies try to reproduce the estrogen they're losing. Estrogen is stored in fat, which is why in midlife many of us start to gain weight, especially in our middle.

It was a relief to know that the invasion wasn't necessarily unnatural. Now when my mother told me I needed to lose weight, I could bark back with confidence that I was in menopause and this was what my menopause looked like.

As I was going through this process of awareness, there was increasing research reported on the hazards of carrying fat around the stomach. Even if you are otherwise thin, it increases the risk of diabetes, heart disease, and Alzheimer's. The Alien was not only unsightly but also dangerous, a relief for you gals fretting about large thighs or upper arms that jiggle. Was liposuction or a tummy tuck the answer? These procedures may decrease superficial fat, but not the negative health impact of these particular fat cells.

I NEEDED TO RETHINK THE HEALTH OF MY ENTIRE BODY, rather than fixate solely on the Alien. I hate taking pills, but committed myself to a daily multivitamin and calcium supplements for general health and bone strength. My skin has always been dry, and I knew it would inevitably become drier with these hormonal changes. Shelley, a former book editor of mine, is a few years older, yet has the dewy skin and shiny hair of someone several years younger. She swears it's because of the massive doses of Norwegian fish oil she consumes. I've since set these capsules out in a small bowl prominently placed on my kitchen counter and pop them like candy. When I'm vigilant, my skin does feel smoother to the touch.

I was raised to believe that relying on prescription drugs rather than the sheer force of will was a personal defeat. Nonetheless, I took my doctor's advice and went on Crestor, a statin, to lower my cholesterol; Advair and Singulair to treat the bit of asthma I developed during this seemingly endless body and life transition; and Wellbutrin, an antidepressant, to cope with the anxiety of it all. Ultimately, my goal is to wean myself from this money pit, but I needed their help to move on and start healing. I wanted to get stronger physically and emotionally.

In "The Melanoma Letter" published in 2004 by the Skin Cancer Foundation, Dr. Marie-Franc Demierre of the Boston University School of Medicine describes growing evidence for statins as a protector against melanoma. Despite the benefits of statins, however, they also tax the liver. Every decision we make in life is a trade-off. Considering my long history of sun abuse, I'm betting the benefits outweigh the negatives.

I had always been a walker, which along with hot yoga helped me stay grounded through my divorce, but now I wanted to shake my body up with more awakenings. I joined the local Y and bumped up my aerobics with a new class they offered called Zumba, a Latin American hip-hop dance workout that not only way ups the endorphins—those feel-good hormones that trigger our opiate receptors—but is also fun and feels sexy. Each session flies by as quickly as the calories burned, which are considerable—allegedly between four hundred and eight hundred an hour.

I WANTED STRONGER LUNGS. My sisters' and my lungs are showing signs of wear—theirs with pneumonia. One smokes, the other never has, yet we were all subjected to the ill effects of our dad's cigarette addiction. I trusted that aerobics would rejuvenate my lungs.

I WANTED STRONGER BONES to slow down any forms of osteoporosis that may be itching to kick in. My youngest sister has osteopenia, an indication of low bone density.

I WANTED STRONGER MUSCLES. Strong muscles meant a stronger body, which means more freedom. I started lifting weights after learning its benefits to building both bone and muscle strength, and how, unlike aerobics, it keeps the metabolism revved in high gear for hours after a workout.

I WANTED A STRONGER CORE to lessen the possibility of back injury. I had begun to hold myself differently since the Alien appeared, much like a pregnant woman compensates for her growing stomach. A stronger core might keep my back in check. I started going to an occasional Pilates mat class, which I found incredibly difficult. I knew not to chastise my body when it couldn't keep up, but to keep at it until my brain and muscle memory became acclimated.

By paying attention to my body in a hands-on physical way, I began to develop a new appreciation for its strengths, vulnerabilities, and potential. Health was becoming my new vanity. I gradually replaced the worn, faded tees, tanks, and workout pants that had been unfortunate stepchildren in my closet with sleek active wear that fit better (thank you, Lycra), and helped me move more comfortably (thank you, Lycra). I liked what these clothes said about me: *I'm active, I'm taking care of my body and I'm proud of it!* I got excited about what was next, until I remembered the rest of my closet.

As I struggled to find my own answers to *How should I look?* I realized that I also needed to think about how I wanted to feel. I needed to start treating myself with loving kindness, which meant not beating myself up every day when I faced my closet, but I also didn't want my clothes to make me look pregnant when I wasn't. I wanted jeans that fit. I no longer wanted to surround myself with anything or anyone that made me feel bad about myself, including my closet.

So after years of failed New Year's resolutions, forsaken diets, whining about my body and now closet betrayal, I decided to crowd out the negative with positive actions and thoughts. Practically applied, drinking more water and green tea meant drinking less coffee and wine. Filling my kitchen closet with healthy foods meant less opportunity to eat junk. Exercising more meant an increase in endorphins and, please God, a decrease in weight. Spending more time with inspiring, feel-good people meant less time for negative, feel-bad people. More gratitude meant less griping. You get the idea. I needed this kind of attitude shift toward my closet.

The Assess, Dejunk, and Renew process that I had sworn by since I took control of my closet decades ago was now too depressing to undertake. I was not about to discard all of the "me" that no longer fit. Rather than focus on negatives—a closet filled with beautiful clothes that still belonged to a younger woman—I unceremoniously shoved things aside to make a little space for *feel-good clothes only!* There had to be a few I owned.

This was the start of my Feel-Good Closet.

7

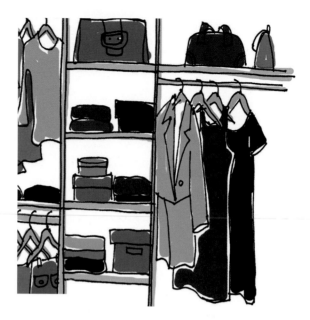

The Feel-Good Closet

I spit on my closet every time I pass it. I'm more spiritual than ever, but my clothes aren't following the spiritual path I am. They draw me back to earth.

—Ali, thirty-nine, Feng Shui consultant, Brooklyn, New York

A Feel-Good Closet is simply a space within your closet reserved for the clothes you *feel* good wearing. It might not be much, but it's a start—a really good start in revitalizing your friendship with your closet. And like all good friendships, a Feel-Good Closet is a safe haven devoid of judgment. To start your Feel-Good Closet, it's important to turn a deaf ear to the fashion police, your mother, children, husband, or anyone else with an opinion, even if you value it. Only you can know if something physically and emotionally feels good to wear. If you second-guess your feel-good choices by worrying what others might think, you'll drive yourself nuts.

Much like everything else about you, your Feel-Good Closet will be unique. Some women aren't comfortable unless they're wearing a bargain with bragging rights. Others don't feel worthy unless their closet is dominated by pricey designer brands. Some dress to fit in, others to stand out. Your Feel-Good Closet may be mixes of comfort clothes, power clothes, and clothes you simply feel pretty in. The sweatpants you enjoy relaxing in may be as important to you as the red cashmere sweater you feel sexy wearing. There is no hierarchy to their value. They each hold their own in your Feel-Good Closet.

I was a guest style expert on a celebrity talk show featuring a segment on makeovers. My assignment was to dress a beautiful woman just released from a hospital, where she was being treated for bulimia, in clothes that would enhance her body, rather than the baggy sweats she hid in. She looked terrific in everything I had her try on, but didn't feel good about her body yet and lacked the confidence to bare any of it. She ended up wearing pearly white silk flowing pants with a matching tunic and an over-vest, which looked ethereal. More importantly, these were clothes she felt comfortable in.

Only you can determine what makes you feel good. If you like wearing your velvet stretch pull-on pants, don't reject them just because your girlfriends have decided that elasticized waistbands are the first sign of losing it—"it" being your figure and your youth. Simply wear tops that cover the waistband and never ever wear a shirt tucked in. If you feel bad about the size of a garment that otherwise flatters—cut the size tag out and forget about it. A good fit will help you feel better about yourself however much you weigh. If you're in doubt, leave those pieces hanging elsewhere. The goal is to create a space within your closet where you can find whatever it is that helps you feel your best this very minute.

And for some, setting aside space for a Feel-Good Closet becomes an awareness of early closet influences.

For many of us, creating a Feel-Good Closet is a necessary step in the process of redefining our self-image—learning to dress from the inside out.

> "The months before I turned forty, I wrote down forty things to do within three months after turning forty. It made this milestone more of a project. Not big-deal changes like skydiving, but more manageable things like getting control of my closet. I finally love my closet. I have carefully edited it down to black, gray, brown, white, and denim solids with an occasionally leopard print or python texture thrown into the mix. I find it liberating."
>
> —*Sara, forty, publishing entrepreneur, Chicago*

At the memorial service for the Japanese-born jewelry designer Kazuko, video clips were shown of her appearing in several Robert Frank movies and in *Six Degrees of Separation*. She was beautiful, arresting, and—most startling to me—dressed in black. In the thirteen years I had known her, she only wore white. There had been a moment in her life when she decided that what she wore was vital to her physical and emotional health, so she created a Feel-Good Closet. For her that meant only wearing white. She believed black weakened inner organs. She also stayed clear of tight clothing, which she felt restricted positive energy. And she created an unbelievable universe of positive connections for the women and men who wore the healing jewelry she made by hand.

Your Feel-Good Closet is a place of certainty, however small, within an abundance of confusion. It's the base camp for your journey to discover what you want to wear for the rest of your life. Like a French woman, you don't need a lot of stuff in your closet, just the right stuff.

Instant Benefits of a Feel-Good Closet

Finding the feel-good clothes you already own is like seeking the comfort of old friends when you need them most. It's what makes your Feel-Good Closet a place of refuge.

Getting dressed will be a lot quicker and easier, because the clothes you enjoy wearing are easy to locate.

By grouping feel-good clothes together, you'll start wearing them more frequently, and with one another in new ways.

Your Feel-Good Closet is within your budget, because you already own what you choose to put in it. In the process, you'll likely discover clothes you hadn't thought of wearing in a while, perhaps because they needed tailoring or were missing an accessory like the right shoes or a flattering undergarment—or maybe you simply forgot they existed, because you couldn't see them.

Your Feel-Good Closet is flexible. Some items will always be ready to serve, while others might eventually commit treason, and there will be those that simply change from one season to the next.

Your Feel-Good Closet will help you recognize the common elements— color, style, texture—of the clothes that you enjoy wearing, which will make shopping for your Feel-Good Closet feel less overwhelming.

Starting your Feel-Good Closet gives you the opportunity to organize that part of your closet space more efficiently.

Your Feel-Good Closet is a source of confidence. It is your fresh start in redefining your self-image.

What's in a Feel-Good Closet?

- Clothes that fit and flatter your body, whatever its size.
- Clothes that are comfortable to wear.
- Clothes that help you feel the way you want to feel.
- Clothes that give you confidence.

When you are clothes-confident, you will feel more body-confident, which will help you feel more life-confident.

8

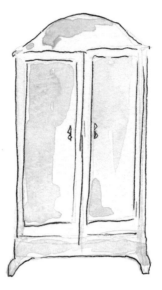

Beginner's French

For more than a decade early in my career as an editor at *Town & Country*, *Avenue*, and *Esquire* magazines, I had the privilege of covering the fashion collections in Paris for several weeks a year. What was displayed on the runways was exciting to observe, although way out of reach given most of our lifestyles and bank accounts. What I always found more intriguing was roaming the streets and observing French women in everyday life. Whatever their status, shape, size, or age, they looked terrific in what they wore.

> *Dressing is a way of life.* —Yves Saint Laurent

FRENCH WOMEN ARE LEGENDARY FOR PACKING THEIR STYLISH WARD-ROBE INTO ARMOIRE-SIZE CLOSETS. For centuries, the limited space taught them that to stow a chic wardrobe required discipline, self-scrutiny, and mindfulness. However small or large their closets may be today, as a culture they continue to abide by those principles that have made French style indisputably renowned.

FRENCH WOMEN DRESS TO PLEASE THEMSELVES. The French may have invented fashion, but French women are not slaves to it. They treat it with respect and appreciation; they know to take from it only what they personally enjoy wearing and ignore what doesn't suit them.

We must never confuse elegance with snobbery.
—Yves Saint Laurent

FRENCH WOMEN ARE SCRUPULOUS ABOUT WEARING CLOTHES THAT FIT PERFECTLY. It's not uncommon for them to have even the cheapest garment tailored to fit their body better.

FRENCH WOMEN KNOW THAT QUALITY IS MORE IMPORTANT THAN QUANTITY. A French woman would rather blow a month's salary on a fabulous suit that she'll wear five days a week in varying ways than share the precious real estate in her armoire with clothes she doesn't enjoy wearing, whatever their cost. In contrast, despite the fact that the American closet averages fifty square feet, and the footage of rentable self-storage units increased by 740 percent between 1985 and 2007, a common lament of American women is "I have a closet full of clothes and nothing to wear."

Lise, a fifty-four-year-old partner in a law firm, is addicted to finding a deal. Consequently her closet is packed with clothes, many of which don't fit. "I hate my closet. There's too much stuff and I can't seem to throw any of it out. A lot of things are wrinkled because they are crushed, and often I can't find pants that go with a jacket."

Lise is not alone.

FRENCH WOMEN KNOW THAT "CLOSET CLASSICS" ARE A WARDROBE'S SECRET WEAPON. They will save you money and will often save your derriere. They will help you build a closet with care and awareness so you are ready for anything. What are Closet Classics? They are a gal's best friends. Jeans, a black dress, a well-tailored suit in a neutral color, a white shirt, a cashmere sweater, black pants—they're the clothes that you constantly reach for and that never go out of style whatever your age. They mix easily with fashion whimsies and other wardrobe favorites to suit your mood and the occasion. And most importantly, you can always rely on them, because they are always appropriate.

FRENCH WOMEN KNOW THAT A FEW CLOSET CLASSICS AND ACCESSORIES ARE THE WORKHORSES OF THEIR CLOSET. By mixing and matching them, they transform a small armoire into a huge wardrobe. French women might wear the same black pants or charcoal skirt for days, but simply change a scarf or a jacket—and *voilà!*

A woman's wardrobe shouldn't change every six months. You should be able to use the pieces you already own and add to them. Because they are like timeless classics.

—Yves Saint Laurent

FRENCH WOMEN KNOW THAT ADDING A SOUPÇON OF SURPRISE to what they wear makes their style distinctive. It might be the coquettish flounce of a skirt, a flurry of fabulous faux jewelry, or a splash of a surprising color.

FRENCH WOMEN KNOW THE POWERFUL CONNECTION BETWEEN WHAT THEY WEAR AND HOW THEY FEEL, so they take delight in dressing whether they're alone, shopping for groceries, or out on more special occasions.

I don't understand why someone would leave the house without fixing herself up a little—if only out of politeness. And then, you never know, maybe that's the day she has a date with destiny. And it's best to be as pretty as possible for destiny. —Coco Chanel

FRENCH WOMEN KNOW THAT COMFORT AND STYLE ARE SIMPATICO, although they can enjoy the fun of wearing a pair of naughty shoes when they don't have to walk.

FRENCH WOMEN ARE NOT YOUTH-OBSESSED. They dress to honor the women they are and bodies they have at any age.

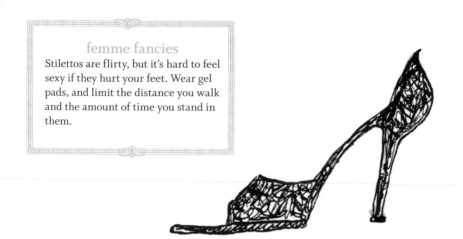

You can only perceive real beauty in a person as they get older. —Anouk Aimée

FRENCH WOMEN ARE NOT HESITANT TO DRESS TO EXPRESS THEIR FEMININITY, SENSUALITY, OR SEXUALITY.

A mature woman in Europe is considered sexually powerful.
—Catherine Deneuve

FRENCH WOMEN TAKE COMFORT IN WHAT THEY WEAR.

To be beautiful, all a woman needs is a black pullover and a black skirt and to be arm in arm with a man she loves.
—Yves Saint Laurent

FRENCH WOMEN CARRY THEMSELVES WITH CONFIDENCE, which translates into great posture, which makes everything they wear look better.

Look for the woman in the dress. If there is no woman, there is no dress. —Coco Chanel

9

Finding Your Feel-Good Closet

The only obstacle between you and your Feel-Good Closet, if you allow it, is your relationship with your mirror, your underwear, and yourself.

Step 1. Why Wait to Look Great?

Closet Confidential: Wear to Start

"I've never felt comfortable dealing with clothes because I didn't have a flair for them. It was easier to ignore the issue and look like I didn't care, rather than try and fail. Besides, I was someone who had always relied on being attractive. That's been the toughest part of aging. So much of my self-esteem had been fueled by the way people reacted to my looks. I want to age gracefully, but I really do care a lot about how I look. Now I'm trying to dress better for my body, so I feel better about myself."

Francesca, fifty-two, Edina, Minnesota

Don't put off finding your Feel-Good Closet with excuses. "Why bother? Nobody cares," "I don't have the time," "I don't have the money," "I don't know where to start," and the most common, "I'll start when I lose weight."

> All research to date on body image indicates that women are much more critical of their appearance than men, likely because they are more judged on their appearance. The constant exposure to idealized images of female beauty on television, in magazines, and in advertising makes exceptional good looks appear to be the norm, and anything short of this perfection seem abnormal or even ugly.

The process will be gradual. You're going to shop your closet before spending a dime, and trust me, unlike men, women are wired to always feel they need to lose weight, so get over it! When you berate your body, you will never feel good in anything you wear. And let's face it: Most of us are obsessed with at least one aspect of our body—jowls, patches of cellulite, wrinkles, jiggly arms, disappearing derriere, drooping eyelids, sagging breasts, graying hair. Just as we come to terms with what we feel is one glaring flaw, we find another to complain about. Today women are even having cosmetic surgery to reduce the size of their clitoris, and often with their daughters! We each have our Achilles' heel if we allow it.

> According to *TIME* magazine the number of women in the United States getting genital cosmetic surgery increased 20 percent from 2005 to 2006; in the UK, it doubled between 2002 and 2007. And for the first time, a US medical textbook on women's reproductive health published in 2009 included a chapter devoted entirely to female genital plastic surgery.

And don't worry about feeling pressured to ditch any of your clothes unless you choose to. Finding your Feel-Good Closet is not having to let anything go, but simply placing together the clothes you feel great wearing in a designated space. Everything else is backup.

When you wear the clothes that occupy your Feel-Good Closet, you will look and feel better about yourself every time you face the mirror. It simply takes a commitment and an awareness to honor your body by dressing to flatter it.

So why wait to look great?

Step 2. Bird by Bird

Rather than analyze your entire closet in one sitting, let's start with a series of baby steps, or what I like to call "bird by bird"—the title of Anne Lamott's inspiring book on the writing process. Lamott tells a childhood story of how panicked her brother was when he realized his school report on birds was due the next day and he hadn't started working on it. Their father advised him not to think of the bigness of the assignment, but to simply write about one bird at a time—bird by bird.

I often think of this wisdom when anything in life threatens to be overwhelming. So rather than being daunted by the task of dejunking your closet to make room for your Feel-Good Closet, just clear a small area to house it—some hanger space, a drawer, and part of a shelf is ideal. If you need storage space, consider purchasing a few clear plastic drawers that can be placed on the floor of your closet or under your bed. One woman I interviewed stored hers under tables covered by floor-length fabric.

Clearing out some space for your Feel-Good Closet also provides an opportunity to rethink your closet organization. One woman lined a small guest room with cedar planks and set up portable clothing racks to make room for her Feel-Good Closet. Another wallpapered hers. What's important is that everything you include in your Feel-Good Closet be easy to see.

Step 3. Mirror Talk

Your mirror can be your friend or your foe, and unlike the one that belonged to Snow White's wicked stepmother, it's not always honest. Out of habit we generally see in the mirror only what we want to. We stand a little straighter, hold our heads a little higher, and pull our tummies in a little tighter. Most of us know from experience how deceptive our perceptions can be. A chance glimpse of ourselves off-guard or an unflattering photograph can catch us by surprise.

As Joan Didion describes in *The Year of Magical Thinking,* her book about the sudden death of her husband:

> Marriage is not only time: it is also, paradoxically, the denial of time. For forty years I saw myself through John's eyes. I did not age. This year for the first time since I was twenty-nine I saw myself through the eyes of others. This year for the first time since I was twenty-nine I realized that my image of myself was of someone significantly younger.

Mirror Talk is a series of reality checks that will help you learn to use the mirror as a constructive tool. It may not be a friend, but it's definitely an expert witness. With time you will develop a critical eye, and the dialogue between you and your mirror will become second nature.

To start, you need a full-length mirror and a large handheld mirror so you can take a good look at what you're wearing from all angles, and lighting bright enough to see subtleties like contrasting colors or bulges. I am all for living life in the most flattering lighting available, but I have experienced the dread of knowing that a bad clothes day was ahead of me when racing from home to a meeting only to discover that I was wearing grotesquely different shades of navy or socks that differed in color.

Ali, thirty-nine, a Feng Shui consultant, navigates her full-length mirror on wheels to assess the overall effect of what she is wearing in soft, forgiving light before angling the mirror to check details in the harsher light of reality. But she admits in exasperation, "I say things to myself when I look in the mirror that I wouldn't even say to my worst enemy." What is important about Mirror Talk is not to be judgmental about your body, but to focus only on how the clothes you are wearing look on your body.

If you have trouble facing the mirror, put on some happy mirror music. A University of Toronto study published by *Prevention Magazine* showed that volunteers were better able to solve challenging word puzzles after thinking happy thoughts and listening to upbeat music. Conversely, serious moods and sad music limited their ability to think outside the box.

MIRROR MUSIC

"Respect Yourself" by Luther Ingram and Mack Rice
"I Won't Back Down" by Tom Petty and Jeff Lynne
"I Will Survive" by Freddie Perren and Dino Fekaris
"Dream a Little Dream of Me" by Fabian Andre and Wilbur Schwandt
"I Feel Pretty" by Leonard Bernstein and Stephen Sondheim
"I'm Too Sexy" by Richard Fairbrass, Fred Fairbrass, and Rob Manzoli

W2W Closet Journal: Friendly Mirror

It's time to start a W2W Closet Journal—a notebook where you can keep track of the practical, the inspirational, and your feel-good priorities as you reshape your closet.

When you look in the mirror, acknowledge that you love yourself. Just do it! Then tell yourself what you like about your body. Long eyelashes, shapely ankles—anything! Be gentle as if you were talking to your daughter or a good friend. If you drift into negatives, tell yourself out loud to stop, then refocus on the positive.

Write your "assets" down. Date it.

Caring Closet

Lighten up! If lighting is a problem in your closet, Bed Bath & Beyond offers a variety of stick-on bulbs that don't require wiring, tools, or an electrician.

Step 4. Bare Necessities

What you wear under your clothes is more important than the clothes. It can make what you wear look its best or its worst. I hate wearing underwear (one good thing about my breasts is that they are gravity defying), but what I hate more is wearing clothes that don't sit well on my body, making me feel bad about my closet and myself. As you go through your closet, you'll find you own plenty of clothes that you might not include in your Feel-Good Closet because you aren't wearing the right underwear.

There are essentially four types of underwear:

SEXY LINGERIE is a way of expressing your sexuality, even if no one else knows you're wearing it. They feel empowering to Ruth, a forty-two-year-old attorney in New York City. "A friend told me I should get fitted for a new bra because it changed her life, so I went to a lingerie boutique (La Petite Coquette in New York City) and bought three very sexy bras and panties for more money than I normally spend. I feel totally hot wearing them."

PLAIN JANES are simple, utilitarian, and usually in cotton. They're the closet's equivalent of comfort food, and they feel especially good to wear when you're just relaxing.

ATHLETIC UNDERWEAR is designed to comfortably yet firmly hold in place your breasts and everything else that jiggles when exercising.

BODY SHAPERS do just what you'd think: They hold you up, hold you in, and smooth things out, giving your body its best shape. Although you might feel like a stuffed sausage wearing some of these underpinnings, you will look trimmer and perkier, and your clothes will appear more flattering. When it comes to body shapers, there are many times I sacrifice comfort to look in the mirror and see that everything appears in place and somewhat in proportion.

For you women who have remained trim and fit, and have dodged an Alien—Oprah calls hers "the brown elephant in the room"—Carmen, seventy-seven, a world-famous model, explains, "It's those five pounds that always seem to slosh around." It may be time for you to give yourself a boost with undies designed to prevent just that.

There is room for all types of underwear in your Feel-Good Closet. Your needs will vary depending on activities, body demands, mood, and the particular clothes you wear. Likely you will choose to wear combinations of varying kinds—maybe a sexy bra and body-shaper bottom, or a bra minimizer with cotton briefs. For me, athletic bras are a daily necessity. When I need to "dress," I wear high-waisted body-shaping panties to smooth me up to my breasts, along with a push-up bra that gives me cleavage, which I never had before, and to detract attention from the Alien.

Mirror Talk: Underwear Fit

Each time you put on an undergarment, recheck its fit. Not only is your body evolving, but underwear also stretches out with use, and it may no longer be giving you the support and clean lines you need under your clothes.

When was the last time you changed the size of your bra? According to Neiman Marcus, 80 percent of us are wearing the wrong bra, and the average woman will wear six different bra sizes in her lifetime.

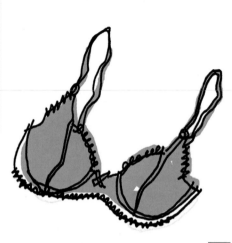

> ### size matters
> Nothing will make you look older than droopy breasts. Be sure your bra gives them a lift. Resize your bras as you lose or gain weight, and pay attention to their condition—they stretch over time. Closet Classics: nude, black, or white bras. Strapless are the most versatile.

Closet Confidential: New Bra, New Life

"The best things I bought recently were new bras. They have changed my life. I wasn't happy with those I had been wearing so I made an appointment with a specialty store (Bra Smyth in New York City) and got fitted. Apparently, I had been wearing the wrong size. The cups were too small and the straps were too big. I was so happy with the change that I threw out all my old bras."

Terry, forty-six, financial consultant, Manhattan

If your bra no longer gives you a lift, junk it. Giving your breasts a boost with a proper-fitting bra will help your body look younger and sleeker. The wrong fit can cause muscle tension and back problems.

Bras should not be noticeable unless intentional. They are best when soft, comfortable, seamless, and smooth, yet durable enough to support and enhance.

Bra cups should caress rather than squeeze your breasts, causing overflow. Nor should they be roomy, causing a visible gap.

The bra band accounts for 90 percent of breast support. If your bra rides up in the back, the bra band has likely stretched out. If it accentuates back flab or if the space between the cups doesn't lie flat, go up a size.

> ### Closet Confidential: *Reality Check*
>
> A very fit forty-six-year-old mother I talked with was startled when a closet consultant suggested that she start wearing Spanx. "I am trim, active, and frankly didn't think I was old enough to wear body shapers, because I have a three-year-old son. But the consultant was right. I had no idea that my back needed a little ironing out."

If cellulite, waist flab, droopy butt, flabby stomach, or panty line is noticeable, you need a change in panties.

Keep watch for pinched flesh. It's not only unseemly, but also indicates that you need to size-up your panties or wear those that are laser-cut rather than elasticized at the trim.

SHOP SMART: UNDERGARMENTS

If your underwear isn't doing its best job, put it on your Shop Smart shopping list. Your Feel-Good Closet can benefit if you add a few key undies. Boutiques that specialize in undergarments and large stores like Nordstrom have trained sales experts who are current in new product developments and can help you determine your fit. Make an appointment in advance of your shopping trip.

If you need some smoothing out under a particular pair of pants or a knit top, take them with you when shopping.

Don't get stuck on size. Your underwear must fit you; you don't fit into your underwear. Sizing varies with manufacturers and with styles.

Don't assume you know what works best for you. Experiment! There are manufacturers like NuBra, Sassybax, and Spanx committed to improving the design, technology, and fabrics of undergarments, providing us with more flattering options for our particular body and clothing needs.

. . . FOR BRAS

Make sure your bra fits firmly on the center hook.

If one breast is larger than the other, go with the larger size and adjust the strap.

Underwire bras provide support, making for perkier-looking breasts.

If you have full breasts, silicone gripping tape and firm cups will help hold them in place. "Minimizers" can suppress your bust a complete size.

Padded push-up bras enhance cleavage. There are some with silicone inserts for fuller-looking breasts.

If you prefer not to wear a bra, reusable silicone pasties comfortably mask nipples.

If you need support when wearing backless or strapless clothes, lightweight, self-adhesive silicone bra cups make it possible.

Athletic bras come in varying amounts of support. You'll need more control when running than when practicing yoga. What's important is that the bra holds your breasts in place when working out, to prevent damage to your breast tissue. The most comfortable and efficient are made in moisture-wicking fabrics to keep you cool and dry.

. . . FOR YOUR MIDRIFF

For a clean line between your breasts and your waist, look for a control camisole that contours and shapes your middle. Those with a built-in bra will give your breasts support. Some are pretty enough to show off.

To smooth out your stomach and waist, try a body-shaper panty that extends up to your breasts, pulling in while smoothing out.

. . . FOR BELOW THE WAIST

Thongs guarantee no rear panty line. Some styles offer stomach control.

When pinching is an issue, laser-cut panties are a great alternative to those with an elasticized trim, which can be visible in fitted clothes.

To smooth out cellulite, there are varying lengths of long-legged shapers to give tone to thighs and derriere.

If your butt needs a boost, there are panties designed to lift, and those that are padded to enhance, which is especially helpful if your pants are becoming baggy in the butt.

. . . FOR YOUR OVERALL BODY

For shape and control, body-shaping slip dresses and bodysuits in lightweight fabrics that breathe and wick away moisture comfortably do the job. Strapless versions and those with underwire support are available.

Caution: Before heading out wearing any new underwear, wear it around your home under your clothes while sitting, bending, reaching, and moving for at least half an hour to check for comfort and any possible slippage.

Step 5. Beginner's Closet

The first things to put into your Feel-Good Closet come from shopping your closet, rather than a trip to the mall.

Think French woman's closet. You don't need a lot of options in your Feel-Good Closet. The immediate goal is to find just one great look for each of your everyday activities that you feel comfortable and confident wearing.

W2W Closet Journal: Assess Your Needs

Write your immediate what-to-wear priorities in your W2W Journal: the activities that you dress for in your everyday life.

Date _____ / _____ / _____

_____

_____

_____

_____

Next, get into your closet to find what you need. If what to wear to work is a priority and you prefer wearing pants for the job, start by trying on all the appropriate candidates. When you find a pair that appears suitable, have an honest dialogue with your mirror.

Initially this step requires more time and emotional energy than it will after you have found a few trustworthy items to place in your Feel-Good Closet. It can be especially time consuming at the beginning of a season as you discover that some of the clothes you wore last year might not fit as well. Be patient, and don't attempt to tackle all your wardrobe solutions at once or you will become overwhelmed. Start slow—"bird by bird."

Mirror Talk: Pants

- *Do I like the way these pants make me feel?*
- *Do they fit?* Sit, bend, and walk around for at least thirty minutes before checking in with your mirror—front, side, and rear—without sucking in your stomach or standing taller.
- *Do I have camel toe?* This occurs when your pants give way too much definition between your legs.

- *Would a body shaper help these pants look better on me?*
- *Can I move and sit comfortably?*

If you're satisfied, get back into your closet to find a top and shoes to wear with the pants.

Then, More Mirror Talk

- *Does the top I am wearing skim my body or is it too tight?* Check your back!
- Walk around for a few minutes then come back to the mirror. *Has the top bunched up in an unflattering way?*
- *Are my pants too short or too long for the shoes I am wearing?*
- *Do my socks blend in with the color of the pants or shoes?* Unless you are forgoing socks or want attention drawn to your ankles, wear hosiery in the same tonal color as the pants or shoes for a clean, long, elegant line.

If you decide to build an outfit around a special piece of clothing or accessory, same drill.

If you find you need to buy body-shaping underwear to wear an outfit better, write it down on your Shop Smart list, so you remember to take the garment with you when you shop.

Step 6. Fake It Till You Make It

Fake it till you make it! was the rallying cry of an experienced kayaking guide to encourage me to brave white-water rapids. It meant to keep an eye on where you want to go, rather than focusing on the big scary rocks in the water, which would result in a Siren's Song. His wisdom came at the right moment in my life: I was facing more formidable challenges than river rocks. I discovered that his mantra can be applied to many challenges in life, including a closet challenge. You can fake a lot in your closet when you need to.

If you can no longer button your suit jackets or blazers, but can move your arms comfortably, wear them unbuttoned. If they are tailored and shapely, they will still give you shape and pull your look together.

If you can't zip up your favorite skirts, get yourself into the appropriate control panty. Then fudge it by wearing a tailored jacket or a top long enough to hide the unzipped zipper. If the back of your skirt flares out, deflate the telltale sign of your secret by hiking it up in front at the waist, so the back of the skirt lies flat against your butt.

If a skirt is a bit shorter than you now feel comfortable wearing and if letting down the hem is not an option, wear opaque tights in a dark color to blur the perception of length.

If your skirt hangs below your knees or is shapeless, which can look dowdy, have it tailored. Mid-knee is the most flattering length for all women. A straight skirt should give a bit of shape to your derriere and be tapered a bit at the knee.

If your pants reveal traces of cellulite or panty line, or if they appear baggy in the butt because your derriere has diminished, the appropriate body-shaping undergarments can help. If pockets bunch or make you look bulky, cut them out and mend the seam closed for a faux pocket. If you can't button or zip up your pants, do the same thing you'd do with a tight skirt: Wear a top long enough to hide the unmentionable. If your pants pull across the hips, reveal camel toe, or look skintight, or if you can't sit in them comfortably, it's time to find them a new owner. Recycle.

If a sweater fits snugly, revealing unsightly bulges (remember to check your back), rather than ditch it, tie it around your neck for a hit of color and to attract attention away from what lies beneath.

Never, ever disappear in combinations of baggy clothes. They will make you look bigger! Always counter roomy with fitted, or show a little skin—baring shoulders is usually a safe bet for everyone.

Look for clothes in your closet that show off an asset, especially if you're faking something else. If you have great legs but usually wear pants, switch to skirts and dresses. If you have cleavage, show some.

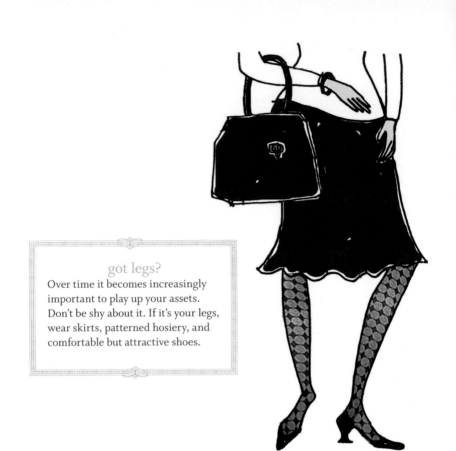

Closet Confidential: A Closet with Legs

"By the time you're fifty, you should know what you have going for you.
It may be your eyes, your hands, or your waist, so capitalize on it! For
me it's my legs. So even in the cold winter months here in Maine when
everyone wears pants, I wear tweed skirts, with patterned stockings and
comfortable shoes with a slight heel. I look great and my husband is
crazy about seeing my legs."

Mary Louise, sixty-something, painter and former fashion editor

Pair monochromatic or tonally colored clothes together to appear thinner
and taller. It will also provide an elegant canvas for eye-catching flour-
ishes of accessories.

Take advantage of your accessories! They will boost your look no matter how much you are faking everything else. And don't save the best only for special occasions. Every day you dress is a special occasion.

Shoes are the quickest fix to polishing your look. Wear those that say what you want them to say—Personality? Style? Quality? Same deal with your bag.

Take a fresh look at your jewelry. Don't be timid. And faux is fabulous. A bold piece can add zip to simple clothes while directing attention away from whatever you're trying to camouflage. I wear a large ring to draw attention away from my weathered hands, and a decorative necklace to bring the eye up and away from my middle.

Fake it till you make it **is knowing that looking good enough is looking great.** You don't want to appear as though you have given up on yourself, but you also shouldn't obsess about attaining "perfection," because nothing in life is ever perfect. For Sally, forty-six, an Australian expat: "Women who look incredibly perfect all the time, in my mind, aren't spending much time on the important things in life, although I think there is a happy balance between the too-casual Aussie style and having everything perfectly in place."

As you continue to shop your closet, your resourcefulness will dissolve frustration into optimism. Self-doubt will be crowded out by confidence.

If you still don't have what you need, write it down on your Shop Smart list.

During my summer of hiding, my priorities were fairly simple. I wanted to camouflage the Alien while wearing:

- Clothes to exercise in.
- Clothes I felt comfortable in during the day while writing or doing errands.
- Clothes or accessories that felt festive to wear when going out with friends at night.

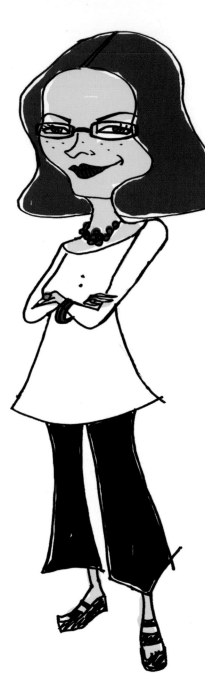

Closet Confidential: Chic in Training

Tessa, a very chic personal trainer in Wayne, Pennsylvania, moves effortlessly through her busy days and nights looking fabulous in exercise pants.

"The trick is to find those that are comfortable, yet don't look like the traditional stick-to-your-skin-show-every-bit-of-trouble exercise pants. They should have room through the legs, be in a sophisticated neutral color—black, brown, dark gray—in a fabric that has some stretch and won't fade. Yoga and Pilates lines are often a good place to find these versatile pants.

"The style of shoes and what you wear on top will change the look from exercise to dining out, not to mention a few bangles and baubles to help jazz things up. This summer I lived in Capri workout pants that I wore under a sleeveless three-quarter-length cotton jersey exaggerated turtleneck, along with fun shoes, gold hoops, and a big faux ivory bracelet. It was a quick throw-on that looked great for art openings, dinner dates, and going out at night with friends."

Caring Closet

Closet karma. For many of us it's hard to let go of clothes that no longer fit our bodies, even when we can't "fake it." There's always the hope it will fit again, or the guilt that it was expensive or received as a gift, or perhaps it holds memories we're not ready to recycle.

Giving your forlorn clothes to others to enjoy as you once did makes it easier. For me, my sisters and daughters get first dibs. Selling to consignment or online shops can supplement a clothing budget. Thrift shops donate proceeds to charitable causes. Find an organization whose mission is to help less fortunate women dress to feel pretty and appropriate. Dress for Success accepts gently worn professional clothes to outfit (and train) women in need of employment. Recycle prom dresses and bridesmaid dresses to one of the many organizations that will provide them to high school girls in need.

I had gradually been adding to my Feel-Good Closet varying styles of cropped black stretch workout pants that could do double duty outside the gym. I wore them that summer under blousy linen shirts and roomy off-the-shoulder tops. The combination comfortably and stylishly diverted attention from my middle while showing off my legs. And I leaned heavily on cheery accessories to boost my morale and add pizzazz to the overall look.

This quick fix got me through the summer feeling comfortable and placated—that is, until panic set in after I received a challenging invitation. Yikes! I needed to get into my closet and look for the white water.

10

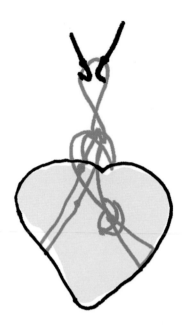

Dressing to Meet My Ex's Next

She's ten years younger than I am. Her last marriage left her with money, two young boys, and, rumor has it, very little body fat. My daughters like her, and she makes their father laugh—he's behaving like the man I fell in love with twenty-seven years ago. Back then, giddy and lovestruck, we felt as if we had won the lottery. Well, he feels that he has won it again. When it came time to meet my ex's next, all I could think was, *What am I going to wear?*

The occasion was a party celebrating our youngest daughter's high school graduation and my ex's fiftieth birthday. For me it marked several major transitions: my becoming an empty-nester, the ex moving on to his next life, and, worst, the status of becoming a "first wife." Needless to say I didn't want to look the part, yet mortgaging my home for a tummy tuck or face-lift was not going to make peace reign within me either.

This moment was about more than looking my best; it was about feeling good about myself and the decisions I had made. I'd never thought that one day I would need to know how to dress like an ex-wife. And what does that look like?

The idea of seeing my ex with his next at my daughter's party brought back memories of what I wore when I met him in college: a blue jean mini skirt, a tight white Hanes boy's tee sans bra, and flat rope-soled espadrilles. A big straw market bag held my books. A cord around my neck was strung with the small white shells I had collected on a beach in Portugal where I'd camped with a friend the previous summer. The Timex strapped to my belt loop measured my life between classes.

During our courtship, I graduated and moved to New York City to work as a fashion assistant at *Town & Country* magazine, while he continued at school. My closet did overtime on a budget straddling my workweek wardrobe and what I wore on weekends visiting him back on campus as the girlfriend of an architecture student. Jeans were uniform for the late-night *charrettes*, when I would assist him in the architecture studio building models or stenciling dimensions onto plans. It was an exciting time of creative support.

> *Charrette* is the French word for "cart." Its meaning expanded in nineteenth-century Paris when architecture students at the École des Beaux-Arts would work furiously on a project until the very last minute, when a cart was literally wheeled through the streets of Paris to collect their submissions to their professors. *Faire une charrette* now means "to be a workaholic," which most architects are.

When he graduated, he left to spend the summer on an architectural tour of Europe. He returned in August with two silver bracelets. It was a special gift, because as he gave them to me, he asked me to marry him. I was thrilled and of course immediately started planning every wedding detail.

My mother was seconds behind along with all her expectations, including what constituted a proper wedding trousseau. No, not sexy lingerie, but a good black dress and a navy blazer: wardrobe basics she felt were the backbone of every stylish woman's closet.

His parents welcomed me into their family by giving me a pearl necklace to which I have since attached a heart-shaped pendant. When given, it represented a classic string of hopes and love that we all shared, this family I married into. That pearl necklace remains a precious part of my closet that I will give to one of my daughters when she marries.

For my wedding, rather than wearing the traditional Cinderella-style gown, I looked as though I was dressed for a *Town & Country* garden story, likely because the *T&C* fashion director designed the dresses that my bridesmaids and I wore. She had been down the aisle a few times before and was over the "princess" dream. To be fair, I had never thought of being rescued by a Prince Charming, so why dress for it? Coming from a long line of Norwegian matriarchs who lived life on their own terms, it was ingrained in me to make it on my own.

It was in May 1981, under sunny skies and a canopy of flowers, that we exchanged vows. I wore a Victorian-style blouse and tea-length skirt in handkerchief linen completed by a wide pink grosgrain sash and white satin ballet flats. Freshly picked baby's breath were tucked into my upturned hair. The overall effect was cinematic—an art director's idealization of a young maiden joyously picking flowers on May Day, a celebration of fertility and spring in many cultures, just before her abduction. Not so far-fetched from reality, however eager a participant I was.

Wearing two pieces rather than a dress suited the practical closet I was gradually filling with clothes that mixed and matched. I thought I would wear my bridal separates forever in varying ways, just as I trusted I would be married forever to this man in all the transformations of sharing a life together. I believed that I could always fit into these clothes and I would never outgrow my dream. But dreams flourish when you're asleep; life happens when you're awake. I outgrew the skirt and sadly, the marriage outgrew us, though not before we shared many years of friendship and love and the gift of having our two daughters in our lives.

We lived as newlyweds in a couple of lofts in Tribeca, which was a quiet-by-night warehouse district in New York City at the time. In the first one, we built the walls with the help of friends; my ex used his architecture prowess to stylishly design the second. Our daughters were born during those pioneer years, before we moved outside the city.

I loved being pregnant and felt fabulous wearing my maternity clothes. My maternity closet held the few pieces I needed for each of those times in my life. Choosing them was an opportunity for a fresh start in creating my ideal wardrobe. Each piece interchanged with perfection. It was like having a suitcase filled with just what I needed for a new adventure—which, of course, becoming a mother was.

Looking back, I can now see how the many closets we shared in our life reflected our unraveling relationship and marriage. These closets were filled with confusion, judgments, and distrust, as we were each also finding our separate ways in life. After so many years of sharing so much, the end came with great sadness. Yet because of our long history together, we found our way back into friendship and became better partners in parenting.

And tonight I was going to meet his next. It was time to dress for me, for my life, and not worry about dressing for him, or even her. Well, maybe a little bit for her. I suspected her curiosity matched mine. I wanted to look glamorous, but I almost screwed it up. With all the stress I felt anticipating this encounter, I had nearly forgotten that it wasn't really about looking a certain way, but about *feeling* a certain way. I needed to look good for me. That's the real special occasion, when you discover how *you* want to feel in what you wear and how you want to behave.

So how do you dress for special occasions that are filled with emotions, insecurities, and expectations? There are a few practical things and a few emotional things to consider beforehand, otherwise you might be stuck with a closet that doesn't even want to be seen with you—the ultimate closet betrayal.

They always say time changes things, but you actually have to change them yourself. —Andy Warhol

W2W Closet Practice: Special Occasions

Respect your closet as you would respect yourself. Never take it for granted. If you don't treat your closet as special, how do you expect it to help you feel special? Your closet can be your friend if you give it the attention and nurturing that all friendships require.

THE PLAN
When I was an editor at *Esquire* magazine, I interviewed Ira Neimark, a seasoned retailer who started his career as a doorman at Bonwit Teller in

New York City and made his way across Fifth Avenue to become the CEO of Bergdorf Goodman. He prided himself on the store's policy: If whatever you bought didn't fulfill your expectations or work with your wardrobe mix when you checked in with your closet, Bergdorf would gladly take it back.

One of the stories he liked to tell was about a fabulously expensive dress that was returned with the sales tags still on along with a peculiar odor. Confounded, he sent the dress out to be tested. The results: formaldehyde. Somewhere in New York, there had been an embalmed woman exquisitely dressed for her final occasion. Agreed, this is an example of extreme closet planning. It's much more fun when you can dress for life occasions and enjoy what you wear for them.

TIMING

So what are your special occasions? They may not be someone else's idea of "fancy," but have special meaning for you. Start a fresh page in your W2W Closet Journal, date it, and list a few of the upcoming events you want to look your best for.

Occasion	Date and Time	Venue	Priority

Always start this process at least four weeks before showtime. If you have a special occasion at the beginning of a season, then make it five weeks. Clothes have a way of looking different from what we remember from one year to the next.

CROSS-CHECK

Before you get into your closet, think about which outfits you can wear to different occasions. For example, do you plan to wear the same suit to a church christening, an afternoon wedding, and the charity lunch you have been invited to? Keep in mind that a change of accessories will vary the look.

PRIORITIZE

Each special occasion has its own urgency. Your priorities have as much to do with timing as with your anxiety. You may decide it's more important to focus on what to wear to your daughter's Bat Mitzvah in four months than to your class reunion in two months.

WHERE AND WHEN

Will the event take place during the day or night, winter or spring, in a ballroom or backyard? What is the dress code? What degree of dressy or casual? If you're not sure, call your host and ask, or find out what the other guests you know will be wearing.

W2W Closet Practice is a good planning tool so you won't be surprised by an event sneaking up on you. It's a good start, but you still need to figure out what you are going to wear. Most of us thought more about what to wear for any occasion when we were sixteen than we do now. We were sensitive to what we wore and how it made us feel about ourselves. Teenage girls continue to try on their clothes (and those of their friends) before going out until they find the right fit for their mood. As years go by, we sometimes lose focus. We forget how special something we wear can make us feel when we put it on, even if we're not feeling so special about our bodies or our lives.

So, what did I want to wear for my eventful night? I wanted to wear something that would help me feel festive. This was an occasion to celebrate my daughter's special graduation. Something distinctive—I was proud to be her mom and I was also proud of the woman I had grown into and the long and special history I had shared with her dad. I wanted to wear something I associated with good memories to bolster my sense of self— something that would make me smile when I put it on. Something that made me feel like a special woman—like me!

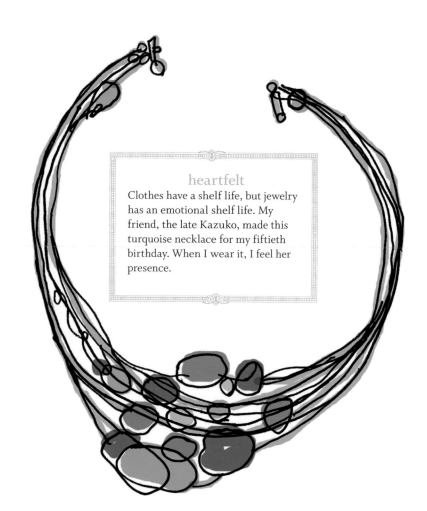

heartfelt

Clothes have a shelf life, but jewelry has an emotional shelf life. My friend, the late Kazuko, made this turquoise necklace for my fiftieth birthday. When I wear it, I feel her presence.

I decided to build an outfit around my favorite necklace—a dramatic turquoise extravaganza that was a fiftieth-birthday gift from a treasured friend. Despite the recent changes in my body, I thought by wearing the right underwear I could find something slimming and sexy from my almost entirely black wardrobe.

As a professional whose career has been advising women on what to wear and personal style, I always recommend preparing well in advance for special occasions. This is rule number one, and I had no excuse not to follow it myself. So why did I ignore my own advice? I suspect it had everything to do with denial.

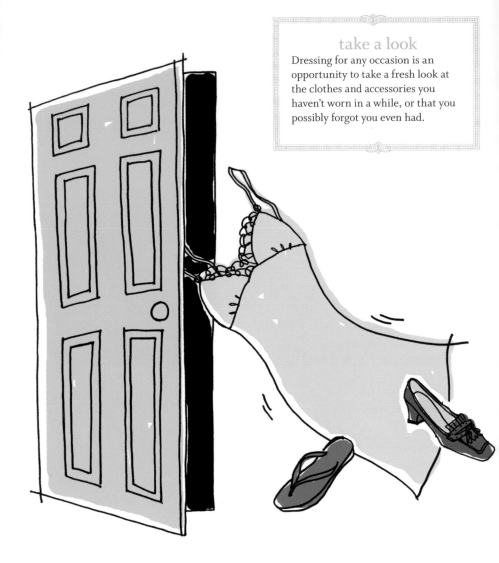

take a look

Dressing for any occasion is an opportunity to take a fresh look at the clothes and accessories you haven't worn in a while, or that you possibly forgot you even had.

W2W Closet Practice (Part 2): Special Occasions

Before getting into your closet, imagine how you want to feel in your clothes—pretty, special, sexy, fun, elegant, naughty, demure? Write down your thoughts in your W2W Closet Journal (page 65) and keep them in mind as you decide what you want to wear. Don't be afraid to reassess.

SHOP YOUR CLOSET

Many women feel they have to shop for special occasions when they might already own something appropriate for the occasion and that looks great on them. Get into your closet, pull out all the possibilities, and try them on—just do it! This is not a time for thinking but one for action. It will also give you the opportunity to dejunk what no longer fits and give you the time to refresh a few things that may need a bit of tailoring. If you're lucky, you may discover a few forgotten treasures that were buried in your closet.

DETAILS

If you remain happy with your discoveries, return to your closet to finish the look. Try on different shoes, bags, jewelry, and a coat or wrap until you find what works to your liking. And remember when spandex was the last thing you put on when getting dressed, not the first? Now your choice of underwear is especially important.

CHECKLIST

If you are missing a few finishing touches, write them down on your Shop Smart list (the worst thing you can do is to shop in last-minute desperation) and get going. Consider bringing at least part of the outfit with you so there is no second-guessing as to what works and what doesn't—save your memory for your friends' names. For example, if you're looking for shoes to go with your navy dress, you'll want to be sure you choose the right tone to match, not clash.

BE SMART

If you need to buy an entirely new special outfit, buy for the weight you are, not the weight you hope to be.

BACK UP

Styles that once looked great on you may now look ho-hum at best, but the opposite can also be true, so always be open to trying on new ideas. Many large department stores provide personal shoppers as a complimentary service with no obligation to buy. Consider a session with one as your very own "style class." Make an appointment and tell the shopper your needs so she can prepare. You may be surprised at the different shapes, cuts, and colors that flatter your body. If the prices are out of your budget, you've at least learned the kinds of styles to look for elsewhere that will be within your means.

PICTURE-PERFECT

Sometimes it's difficult to see the overall effect of an outfit. Ask a trusted and stylish friend for his or her opinion. If you're still uncertain, take a few digital photos for your own assessment. Place the pictures in your W2W Closet Journal or tape them to the wall inside your closet for future reference.

HAPPY DANCE

Don't settle on your outfit until you *feel* the way you had hoped to. Then do what I call the happy dance—even if it's only an inner one. The goal is to look and feel like the best of you.

When I got dressed that evening, nothing worked except for the necklace. The black top I had counted on wearing looked washed-out from wear and, worse, revealed back flab that hadn't been there the summer before. I slipped into a short black dress that had long been a favorite, but it now accentuated the Alien and made my legs look wintry white. The chic black that had always made me look more blond now looked severe. Besides, I didn't want anyone to think I was in mourning. I'm not a widow. I'm an ex-wife! Panic set in as the clock ticked away the minutes I had before I needed to leave. My bedroom was strewn with rejects. There had to be *something* left in my closet that would work.

I am a great believer in buying the basics and then jazzing them up with a few interesting pieces. I've always loved anything in a leopard or a

Pucci-style print. These sexy fashion statements feel fun to wear and can brighten up even the dullest of wardrobes.

With fingers crossed, I reached into my closet and found the stretch Pucci skirt I had splurged to buy (on sale of course) after my divorce. I had justified the cost because wearing it made me feel happy, sexy, independent, and like the me I remembered from what seemed like such a long time ago. Like any true friend, this fabulous skirt had never failed to boost my spirits or forgive my varying weight shifts. Thankfully, it didn't fail me that night. It helped me feel pretty and special.

> Pucci is a distinctive colorful pattern that was first designed by the Florentine aristocrat Emilio Pucci in 1948. Marilyn Monroe loved wearing Pucci's silk jersey dresses as much then as Nicole Kidman does today.

The necklace I had planned to wear didn't work with the end results, but my favorite hoop earrings, a flourish of decorative bangles, gold Jack Rogers sandals, and a black halter top that showed off my arms but hid the back fat and skimmed my middle did. The combination was winning and comforting.

When I looked in the mirror, I was happy to see a composite of who I was at that moment in my life—my daughters' mother, my mother's daughter, a sister, a friend to many, and my ex-husband's ex-wife. I looked like Kim. And most important, I felt great.

My children were pleased with me that night, and my ex seemed proud that I didn't look like "a first wife" even though I was. I was lucky that my closet pulled through. If it hadn't held something I enjoyed wearing, I doubt I would have had the confidence I needed for that transitional life event. I learned never to take any relationship, even that with my closet, for granted again.

Our clothes are a sum of our experiences. We keep those that suit us and should say good-bye to those that don't. I suppose it's a lesson for other aspects of our lives. It takes courage to let go of something that's not working anymore—even after all the mending and tailoring imaginable.

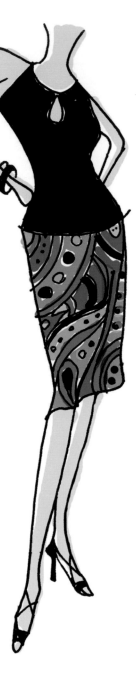

focus

When putting an outfit together,
decide on a focal point that expresses
your mood or suits the occasion. It
might be a piece of jewelry, a festive
print, or decorative shoes. Then build
your look from there.

What I learned from that night is that as much as I know as a style expert, my memory of the clothes in my closet from one year to the next is often brighter than the reality. Special occasions, like objects in the rearview mirror, are always closer than you think. So take heed. When you feel good in your clothes, they become your own special armor.

W2W Closet Journal: Changing Closets

Whether you are dressing for a special occasion or for everyday life, consider how you want to *feel* in your clothes, and think about the ever-changing relationships between you, your closet, and the rest of your life. Write down a few of these thoughts in your W2W Closet Journal.

_____

_____

_____

_____

Closet Confidential: *Moving On*

"I used to pride myself in the elegant and sexy way I dressed professionally and personally," says Michele, a forty-eight-year-old music educator from Alberta, Canada. "But my self-confidence became shattered when I went through an unhappy divorce. I stopped feeling comfortable wearing the beautiful clothes in natural fibers and interesting textures that had made me feel so lively. I started to hide in sweats and yoga pants. I need to move on with my life and regain my self-esteem. I am going to purge my closet and replace it with clothes that will help me feel better about my self-image and dress for a happier life."

To Michele's point, whatever life transition you are moving through, what can be more special than dressing with confidence for a new life—a new you? Now was the time for me to move on in my life—to explore what's next and what I want to wear on this journey.

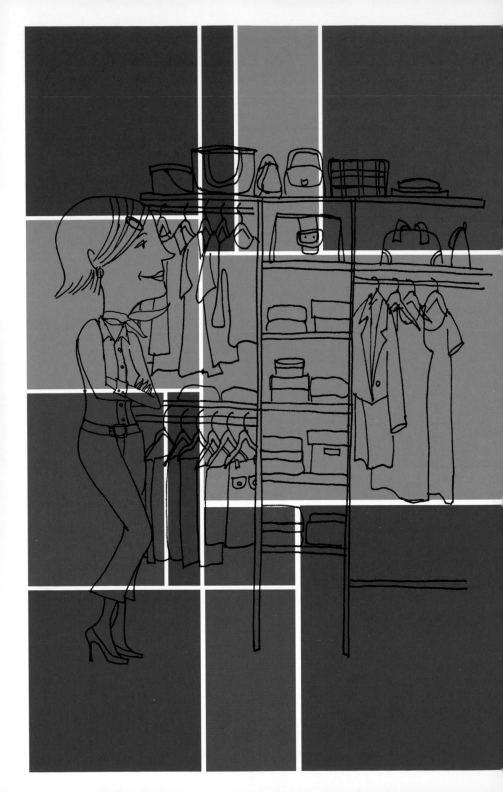

> Our mind is like a parachute, it works when it is open.
> —Dalai Lama

PART TWO
WHAT DO I WANT TO WEAR?

> Without leaps of imagination, or dreaming, we lose the excitement of possibilities. Dreaming, after all, is a form of planning.
> —Gloria Steinem

11

Style Mentors

A magnet on my refrigerator secures a black-and-white photograph of Baroness Marion Lambert. She sits imperiously within the sleek white curves of a starkly sculpted contemporary chair. One leg is tucked under her seemingly fit body while the other folds over her lap. She's wearing a simple black tee, boldly striped zebra-print pants, and black boots. Her head is poised upon her upright arm adorned with two substantial bracelets and a noteworthy pinkie ring. Her blond hair is simply cut to fold just under her clean chin, revealing the large earrings that frame her handsome face. Her commanding presence is softened by light filtered through the tall windows particular to the best addresses in Paris. She looks directly into the camera with an ease that only the utterly confident possess.

I have kept this picture on display at every desk I've worked at since I clipped it out of a magazine when I was a young working girl. To me, she always appeared glamorous and modern despite being several decades my senior. Even the best plastic surgery can't hide the years a neck betrays. She is not a classic beauty, but her style-confidence is compelling. Now that I'm nearing her age in the photograph, I am reminded that style doesn't have to fade with age.

There is an inevitable moment in all of our lives when we can no longer count on the sexual, physical, or lifestyle identity that once defined us. The familiar everyday banter we have with our closets suddenly becomes disoriented as we transition into the next part of our lives. We are no longer merely uncertain about what might be appropriate to wear for an occasion, but what is appropriate to wear for our age.

Closet Confidential: *Style Identity*

"I struggle with my style identity. I'm not yet ready (and I may never be ready) for frumpy old-lady clothes, but fashion for twenty-something-year-olds are not right for me either. I'm confused and stuck and not sure what to wear anymore."

Debreen, forty-five, professional organizer and teacher,
Saratoga Springs, New York

"No one compliments me on how I dress or look anymore. I feel as though I've become invisible."

Ruth, forty-three, Columbus, Ohio

Watching my daughters and nieces as young girls try on a multitude of varying styles in any given day—preppy, hip, Goth, bohemian, and indescribably original—is a wonderful reminder of how clothes were a safe way to try on different identities until we found the right fit.

As we grew into the very busy next part of our lives as worker, wife, mother, friend, and community member, we settled into a style that suited our everyday needs, adding whatever "fashion zip" we felt comfortable with or simply grabbed along the way. Now that we find ourselves in transition once again, many of us lack the style-confidence or know-how to rethink, redefine, and reimagine our self-image. Even as a style expert, I find it easy to get stuck in old style notions that no longer work as well as they once did. The dressing habits we took for granted worked better for another woman—us, in a different time.

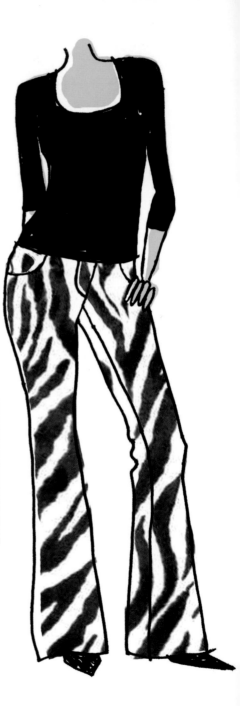

the cat's meow

Animal prints are timeless classics. They add a wallop of chic to the simplest of clothes. But remember, a little goes a long way. Keep everything else you wear with them a quiet neutral.

Baroness Lambert and Karen are just two of the many Style Mentors who have inspired me to reconsider what I want to wear for the rest of my life. I may not live in a luxurious Paris apartment or wear a ransom of jewels as does Lambert, but I love how she combines the elegance of classics with an element of surprise—zebra pants. Perhaps that's why animal prints have long been an important mix in my closet style.

Karen looks fabulous today. There is a joyfulness and confidence in the clothes and accessories she wears, and she wears them with panache. I admire how she had the courage to let go of a memory of who she was and dress to celebrate the woman she has evolved into.

Who are Style Mentors? They are the women we notice. Whatever their shape, height, weight, or age, they wear their style like a second skin. They make the most of the assets they have at the moment. They have figured out what works for them and what doesn't. They wear their clothes with confidence because they enjoy dressing for themselves. They know it's not about trends or necessarily about money, because they don't confuse fashion with style. And they have a reason to get dressed, because they're engaged in life.

I am always on the prowl for Style Mentors—politicians, newscasters, colleagues, women I know or have noticed in passing on the street. Some are legends whose names are synonymous with a look; others are fictional characters in movies, books, or television. Style Mentors show us how to dress to flatter our changing bodies, help us determine what dressing appropriately means to us now, show us how to freshen up our look, and, like Karen, inspire us to dress for the woman we are and the woman we want to be.

My Style Mentors and What I've Learned from Them

Style Mentors are like friendships—each one is unique. One of my Style Mentors is a successful businesswoman about ten years older than me. She reveals her fit arms and legs by wearing skirts or dresses to the knee and sleeveless tops. Beige is her signature color. It brings light to her face and helps her stand out in a crowd of professional women wearing black, at least in New York City. By wearing mules to the office, she declares her personal dress code and her enjoyment of dressing as a woman.

WHY DO I CONSIDER HER A STYLE MENTOR?

I am encouraged that with regular exercise, there's a chance I can be fit at any age. She has inspired me to add colors to my largely black wardrobe, especially those that flatter my face. And like this woman, I enjoy what I wear and am not afraid of dressing like a woman in the workplace, although I am mindful of being appropriate. What inspires me most is that what she wears and how she wears it exude her confidence and self-awareness.

Oprah inspires me in many ways. In terms of style, she shares with us her struggles and triumphs and confusions about her changing body. She shows us that we can dress to flatter our figure whatever its weight. The clothes she wears show off her youthful-looking shoulders, trim waist, and womanly curves. Their colors are as dazzling as her smile is bright, and along with her voluminous soft curls, they enhance her face. I now whiten my teeth, I've softened the look of my hair by having layers cut into what was my signature blunt cut, and I love wearing off-the-shoulder tops. I'm still not comfortable wearing much color, but enjoy it more now as an accent.

Since her debut in the 1977 movie *Annie Hall*, I have watched **Diane Keaton** for style clues much as I would look to an older sister for guidance. I have always admired her individuality, which is reinforced by the unique way she puts clothes together. What she wears doesn't necessarily suit me, but I enjoy her flair and *Why not?* attitude. She dresses for herself. She experiments without worrying about the fashion police.

In the 2003 movie *Something's Gotta Give,* clothes mirror her character's emotional transformation. As a divorced, menopausal empty-nester, successful in her career but bitter toward men, she masked her sexuality behind loose and layered clothes.

> Harry (Jack Nicholson): *I just have one question: What's with the turtlenecks? I mean it's the middle of summer.*
> Erica (Diane Keaton): *Well I guess I'm just a turtleneck kind of gal.*
> Harry: *You never get hot?*
> Erica: *No.*
> Harry: *Never?*
> Erica: *Not lately.*

When her character took the emotional risk of letting herself be aroused by men again (particularly Harry and a younger persistent suitor), she became girlish and celebrated her sexuality by wearing fitted, feminine clothes. Every woman over forty rejoiced in Erica's metamorphosis—we are never too old to feel girlish and sexy, and dress for it.

Diane Keaton is also unique in Hollywood for not attempting to erase years from her life with plastic surgery. At an age when many of us obsess on the subject, she wears her life-lines with a youthfulness that sparkles with her smile, eyes, laugh, and gestures. I am not against cosmetic procedures, but Keaton's example helps me feel more comfortable with my life-lines, too.

In 1972, fashion designer **Diane von Furstenberg** launched her clothing empire with a cotton jersey wrap dress and the tagline *Feel like a woman,* *wear a dress.* The dress remains popular, and the message continues to resonate for women of all ages and body types.

I pay close attention to what DVF wears because we have similar bodies—petite breasts and not much of a waist. She shows off her legs, and bares her shoulders or décolletage with a suggestive frill that directs the eye away from her waist. She looks as sexy, independent, and feminine in what she wears today as she did several decades ago when she appeared on a 1972 cover of *TIME* magazine. And she still enjoys wearing a dress.

Actor and author **Jamie Lee Curtis** has been my hero ever since she appeared in *More Magazine* without wearing makeup, baring her body and refusing to let the photo be retouched. She wanted to let the rest of us girls know that it is okay to age naturally, a radical concept in Hollywood. She continues to pare down her style and possessions by wearing little or no makeup, simple black or white clothes, very few accessories, and a short, no-fuss haircut that does not belie her graying hair. I consider her courageous and cool, honest and humbled, smart and funny, and a great Style Mentor and Life Mentor.

Politicians and newscasters are often great Style Mentors. Their job is to relate to their constituency in an appealing, trustworthy manner, and what they wear is an important way for them to communicate their message. Because they are frequently televised or photographed, they sharpen their style by analyzing what the impartial eye of the camera captures. We can all take a lesson from that.

Meredith Vieira, Diane Sawyer, and Katie Couric all continue to look better with time. Diane has always had light blond hair, but Katie and Meredith have lightened theirs with highlights over the years. They all have softly layered hair, which nicely frames their faces. I always appreciate when they wear their reading glasses on air, a nod to *it's okay, gals—we all need them after a certain age.* And they are all getting a little thicker around the middle, which helps me figure out what shapes are flattering and which ones aren't. And I so appreciate how Meredith has fun wearing color, that Katie shows off her great legs with sexy shoes, and how Diane combines the coziness of a cashmere sweater with the edginess of a leather skirt. Clearly none of their closets are retiring quietly into the next part of their lives.

First ladies represent the women of their country to the world. What they wear serves as a mirror and influencer, so they know to hone their style. Nancy Reagan often wore red, which became known as "Reagan Red"; Barbara Bush's three-stranded pearl necklace became part of her signature look; and despite the stress of being first lady, Laura Bush's regal style looked more effortless over the course of her administration. By comparing pictures of what she wore when her husband was first inaugurated in 2001 with what she wore toward the end of his time in office, you can see how her clothes became better tailored and the fabrics less stiff, moving as gracefully as she did in her busy life. Her colors softened, as did her hair, with delicate highlights and a slightly more layered cut, which brought more light to her face and played up her blue eyes. Each of these elements, as subtle as they may be, helps anyone look pounds thinner and years younger.

There can't be enough said about the influence Jackie Kennedy has had on fashion. **Michelle Obama's** style is as fresh and modern as was Jackie's when she was first lady. She wears classics effortlessly, has a penchant for cardigans rather than structured jackets, wears attractive but practical flat or low-heel shoes, and sports sleeveless sheath dresses that show off her gorgeous, athletic arms—which have us all running to the gym. But unlike most presidential wives, Michelle Obama doesn't depend on a particular designer to define her look. She confidently mixes resources, both high and low, and exhibits her love of color and unabashed admiration for a variety of young American designers. Her upbeat, relaxed style is inspirational, because it feels attainable to all American women.

Candace Bergen also proves how a perky haircut and highlights can give your face a lift. In her role on David Kelley's Emmy Award–winning television series *Boston Legal,* she demonstrates how wearing bold necklaces close to the throat and turned-up shirt collars leads our attention to her attractive face rather than her aging neck. And the tailored jackets she wears give her body shape. You can't go wrong with any of these style solutions. They have attitude and elegance. I have adopted them all.

Madonna is a master of reinventing herself as her life continues to change, while **Gloria Steinem** has kept her trademark long locks, eyeglasses, and the jeans that she claims are "older than most people in the United States." She even wore them when she married for the first time at age sixty-six. I appreciate Madonna's constant self-evaluation and masterful rebranding, and Steinem's ferocious sense of self. I am also envious that she fits into her jeans from decades ago. I, unfortunately, do not, although jeans have long been and continue to be an important part of my closet mix.

The zaftig architect **Zaha Hadid** wears boldly designed clothes and accessories, which make her look as artful as her designs. I admire how what she wears is an important part of her self-expression and calculated style. I, too, have started wearing much bolder gestures—usually a piece of faux jewelry. When my daughter Glenna asked why I wore such big necklaces, I told her a style truth: The bigger you are, the bigger your accessories should be. Of course you need to have the confidence to be noticed.

I look to my contemporary, the author **Amy Tan,** who has a clearly defined cool edge in what she wears. I am jazzed by the seemingly undiminished sexual energy of **Tina Turner** and how she's not shy about dressing for it. It's compelling to watch how the clothes that dancer and choreographer **Judith Jamison** wears move as fluidly as her body. I love the joy the **Red Hat Society ladies** have in dressing up in purple suits and flamboyant red hats—pink for those youngsters under fifty. It encourages me to dress more for the fun of it and certainly more for myself.

These women are only a few of my Style Mentors. All of them refuse to disappear quietly into this next part of their lives. Their sense of style and sense of self are one—an expression of the totality of their lives.

Granted some of the women mentioned have large wardrobe budgets, professional stylists, and dress for quite different lives than I live, but when we look for our Style Mentors we can pick up style clues that will help us each make better decisions in what we want to wear as we define our style in this next part of our lives.

Our Mothers, Our Style

We can't ignore the impact of our mothers on our evolving style. Many women enjoy their mother's style influence, while others are witness to how their mothers have given up on themselves, and they fight not to repeat that defeat.

Closet Confidential: The Mother Closet

"My initial influence would have to be my mother and her friends. They dressed simply, elegantly, and always with a sense of humor and flair. Although when I was in my teens I thought they were way too conservative, so I flirted with bohemian and rebellious looks. Over the years I returned to a more tailored simple style, yet I make sure there is always one component that makes a statement like they did. I also get ideas from my friends, yet some are examples of what-*not*-to-wear, which has been just as important in helping me define and develop my own sense of style."

Tessa, fifty-five, personal trainer, Wayne, Pennsylvania

"My mother's face and body were gorgeous and sexy, but since menopause she became totally plain in her personality and her clothes. No more earrings. No more smiles. No more sex appeal. It doesn't matter how old you are to have sex appeal. I have an eighty-five-year-old friend who is a flirt!

"I hope I don't have my mother's genes. Why did she have to change totally? She thinks she's old and she's only seventy-five, but there is no age limit in keeping a young spirit. It doesn't matter how many plastic surgeries you have if you don't have an inner youthful spirit. I say the affirmation each day: *I am young, beautiful, and full of life!* and I dress to express it."

Doris, forty-nine, construction company owner, Queens, New York

"As attractive as my mother is, she is not my Style Mentor. I have disdain for her obsession and vanity about aging. Because she complains about it all the time, I decidedly do the opposite. Mom takes an hour and a half to get out of the bathroom, so I am out within fifteen minutes. She is almost deaf and will not wear a hearing aid. She chooses style over comfort in her choice of shoes, which has wrecked her feet so she can't walk well. I don't want to hurt mine, so I usually avoid wearing heels even though I'm five foot two."

Francesca, fifty-two, Edina, Minnesota

"My mother (sixty-eight) came to the US from China via Taiwan to go to graduate school. I have many memories of her dressing to go to work and to parties. Other mothers in Fairfield County wore preppy conservative clothes, and the Chinese mothers wore very plain clothing that was boring but very practical and durable. My mother would wear flowing silk pants and heels. She looked fantastic. I loved it. My mother loves red: red gloves, red purse, red Ferragamo shoes, and red accents. She wears red lipstick, as did her mother, my grandmother. They were the lipstick queens. I now like wearing red lipstick, too. When my grandmother died, my mother wrapped her lipstick, earrings, and perfume in her handkerchief and placed it in the coffin as a symbolic gesture so she could look great in the next life. I am positive this would have made my grandmother most happy."

Ruth, forty-two, attorney, Manhattan

I appreciate how my mother always dresses with great flair. She inspires me to put pieces together imaginatively; she's taught me how to navigate thrift shops and bargain-basement racks, and to enjoy dressing for every day, not just special occasions. But mostly she has shown me that style doesn't diminish with age (she's eighty-five years young as I write this). In fact she revs it up, especially when her health is challenged or her spirits need a boost, often quoting Katharine Graham, former owner of *The Washington Post*: "Function in chaos, finish in style."

Women Share Their Style Mentors

Closet Confidential: *Inspired*

"Marlene Dietrich is my Style Mentor. She inspired me to wear one color head-to-toe, so you weren't cut in half. It also makes dressing easier."

Carmen, seventy-seven, world-famous model

"I'm inspired by portraits, women on the street and in readable 'real' fashion places like *Town & Country* and catalogs like Vivre. Today I am wearing an all-white tailored pantsuit and white shirt. None of the pieces were actually bought together, but a portrait I saw of Lauren Hutton taken in 1974 wearing all-white inspired me. I went into my closet and pulled it together in my own way."

Hilary, forty-five, magazine executive, Westport, Connecticut

"When I feel like I'm going too far in a direction, I ask myself, 'What would Audrey do?' "

Kathy, forty-five, interior designer, San Francisco

"It gives me great pleasure putting together outfits every day with the painter Milton Avery's color sense in mind—a lavender coat with a dove-gray beret, peacock sweater, and bottle-green beads. His work has become one of my main style influences."

Janis, fifty-four, literary agent, Manhattan

be inspired

We may have our Closet Classics, but that's no excuse to get stuck in a style rut. Be open to the new. Look around. Ask yourself, *Why does she always look so great?* Is there an element you can adapt to freshen up your wardrobe?

"I have learned more about style since moving to New York from Australia by observing all the incredibly stylish women here. I saw a woman walking down Madison Avenue eleven years ago wearing brown and blue. I was so taken with that color combination that I have adapted it into my wardrobe and into my home. My mother doesn't see it—she reminds me that they were my high school colors in Sydney.

"And I have some English girlfriends who have a simple, interesting elegant summer style—white jeans, Moroccan tops, and great earrings. Dressing like them makes me feel youthful."

Sally, forty-six, environmental fund-raiser, Purchase, New York

"I admire the way Julie Christie and Catherine Deneuve have aged. Neither of these women, who are around my age, looks pinched or plastic. They look modern, having lived, but also smart and feminine. Catherine, being French and therefore constantly tempted by good food, has let herself lose her waistline, so she emphasizes her pretty legs and lovely face and she gets plenty of movie roles still."

Kathryn, sixty-five, writer, Manhattan

W2W Closet Journal: Lessons in Style

Who are your Style Mentors? How do they inspire you?

The Ultimate Style Mentors

Years after their deaths, generations of us continue to look to Jackie Kennedy Onassis and Audrey Hepburn for style inspiration. What makes their look so enviable and timeless?

AUDREY HEPBURN, 1929–1993

Audrey had a boyish figure—skinny, small-breasted, no hips or waist—when she started appearing in films. It was a time when Hollywood celebrated voluptuous pinup girls like Marilyn Monroe and Jayne Mansfield. Audrey knew that to succeed she had to dress to flatter her very different body type: "I tried to make everything an asset. You have to look at yourself objectively. Analyze yourself like an instrument; you have to be absolutely frank with yourself. Face your handicaps, don't try to hide them. Instead, develop something else."

She worked closely with her lifelong friend, the designer Hubert de Givenchy, to create a look that was glamorous and became familiar to us on screen and off. The classics they made famous together include the little black dress—long and short (*Breakfast at Tiffany's*, 1961); the skinny black pant, black turtleneck, and flat black pointy shoes (*Funny Face*, 1957); the fitted white shirt that tied or wrapped at the waist (*Roman Holiday*, 1953); the trench and three-quarter bracelet sleeves (*Charade*, 1963); fitted T-shirts, Capri pants, ballet flats, Sabrina heels, and "décolleté Sabrina" (now referred to as the boat-neck collar), which was designed to play up her shoulders and play down her bony collarbone (*Sabrina*, 1954); and always the silk headscarf and large sunglasses.

Audrey was never trapped by glamour. "I never think of myself as an icon. What is in other people's minds is not in my mind. I just do my thing." She lived and dressed for her life in the present. "I cannot look back with nostalgia at a coat I enjoyed wearing years ago. I was inside it and it kept me warm but I am still here and the coat is something of the past. Or of a photograph of me: I don't look at a photograph of myself fifteen years ago with regret or nostalgia, although I can be amused or fascinated." And she always understood how the clothes we wear can inspire self-confidence. In a note to Givenchy, she wrote, "When I talk about UNICEF in front of the television cameras, I am naturally emotional. Wearing your blouse makes me feel protected."

When she was in her sixties, she divided her time between Ethiopia as a special ambassador for UNICEF, and a home in Switzerland that she shared with her gardens, dogs, and loved ones. Classics remained a part of her wardrobe, but her elegant simplicity evolved, as did her life. She continued to favor slim pants, but they were now more likely to be jeans and khakis. She replaced much of her couture wardrobe with off-the-rack clothing, often designed by Ralph Lauren. Her ballet flats were less likely to be worn, because sneakers, driving moccasins, and garden clogs better suited this time in her life. The fitted white shirts that had wrapped around her waist were sensibly replaced with Lacoste polo shirts and oxford cloth shirts frequently worn untucked. When traveling, she would pull it all together with a well-cut blazer. Her signature gamine haircut grew into her signature French twist, which then became her signature bun. She preferred little or no makeup and rarely wore jewelry.

In 1990, *People* magazine proclaimed the sixty-one-years-young Audrey Hepburn as one of the fifty most beautiful people in the world. Her idea of beauty is ageless: "For beautiful eyes, look for the good in others; for beautiful lips, speak only words of kindness; and for poise, walk with the knowledge that you are never alone."

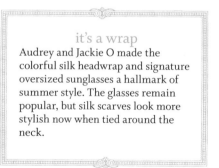

it's a wrap
Audrey and Jackie O made the colorful silk headwrap and signature oversized sunglasses a hallmark of summer style. The glasses remain popular, but silk scarves look more stylish now when tied around the neck.

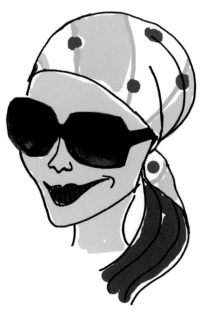

JACKIE KENNEDY ONASSIS, 1929–1994

I am a woman above everything else. —Jackie Kennedy Onassis

What Jackie wore always mirrored the life she led.

No woman in the history of the White House has had more lasting influence on the way women dress than First Lady Jacqueline Kennedy. The retrospective Jackie Kennedy: The White House Years—held at the Metropolitan Museum of Art in 2001, and now largely housed at the Kennedy Center Library and Museum in Boston—displayed evidence that she understood how clothes were a calculable and powerful form of communication and connection, especially as wife of the president of the United States. She collaborated with designer Oleg Cassini to create her White House wardrobe. She wore color to stand out in a crowd and low-heeled shoes for comfort on the campaign trail. She knew how to show off her well-toned arms and legs by wearing sleeveless knee-length dresses when appropriate and suits with discreetly feminine three-quarter-length bracelet sleeves. Substantial pearl necklaces brought light to her face, and her neatly coiffed yet relaxed bouffant hairdo remained her style signature for life.

Evening dresses were designed spectacularly yet with simple, clean lines and pale colors, which allowed her to shine. In 1961, she accompanied her husband to Vienna for tense meetings with then Soviet Premier Nikita Khrushchev, and dazzled the premier at a dinner hosted by the Austrian president with her renowned charm and a pale pink silk georgette chiffon evening dress embroidered with sequins. Khrushchev declared it "beautiful." When he had a photo op the following day shaking hands with JFK, he asked to shake Jackie's first.

It is noted in the catalog from the exhibit curated by Hamish Bowles that rather than wearing the more formal church attire of 1962, which often included hat and gloves, Jackie attended a Good Friday service in Palm Beach wearing Jack Rogers Navajo sandals along with a sleeveless sundress and head scarf. Many across America were offended. "Little did we realize that we would have in Jackie, a sort of beatnik, a gilded one, of course," wrote one outraged citizen.

As Jackie O, she sought privacy on the yacht or Greek island owned by her second husband, Aristotle Onassis. She hid behind huge sunglasses and silk headscarves, which she often wore with large hoop earrings, Schlumberger enamel-and-gold bangle bracelets (still available at Tiffany's), fitted T-shirts, white jeans or Capri pants.

After she turned forty and was widowed yet again, she became an editor at Doubleday in New York City. As working Jackie, her uniform was Valentino's softly draped trousers and silk shirts in warm colors—browns, purples, mauves, lavender, and pinks—a trench coat, and sensible low-heeled shoes for professional chic. Her signature earrings were Schlumberger enamel-and-gold earrings from Tiffany's.

On weekends, she was often seen racing around New York City on her bicycle wearing white jeans, black turtlenecks, and Keds sneakers. And she was a lifelong equestrian—no one looked better in hacking jackets, riding boots, and jodhpurs.

As a grandmother, she was frequently seen in Central Park with her granddaughters, dressed in her signature trench coat, silk headscarf, oversize sunglasses, dark trousers, and forever the practical low-heeled shoes. At the black-tie fund-raisers for institutions she passionately supported, she continued to wear simply cut long dresses, often with elbow-length sleeves and usually designed by Carolina Herrera.

Jacqueline Kennedy Onassis died in New York on May 19, 1994, and is buried next to John F. Kennedy at Arlington National Cemetery.

It's been said that Jackie looked to Audrey as her Style Mentor. Indeed there are similarities in what they wore, but like all stylish women, they each knew how to adapt a look and make it their own. While Audrey's style was considered low-key Hollywood glamour, and Jackie's American *sportif*, they shared a relaxed elegance in what they wore. They clearly loved fashion, but favored simplicity, quality, and comfort over trends. They also understood how to dress for their bodies. Their great posture and demure demeanor made whatever they wore look regal, whether jeans or ball gowns.

Over the years, their style evolved as gracefully as they did. While some clothes remained a constant in their closet, others were replaced by those better suited for their private and public lives. Yet there remained a consistency to each of their styles throughout their lives. These are the clothes that became our classics. They bridged Old World elegance with modernity, a legacy that continues generations later.

Secrets of Style Mentors

Style Mentors choose the clothes they wear because of how they want to *feel* in them.

Style Mentors are aware of what their clothes communicate.

Style Mentors dress to show off their assets and deflect from their not-so-favorite assets.

Style Mentors know that fit and proportion are paramount to their body looking its best.

Style Mentors pay attention to details. They know that the right underwear and accessories can make or break a look.

Style Mentors know a great haircut can give their face a lift.

Style Mentors have found their signature style—a personal uniform, which evolves as their bodies and lives change.

Style Mentors dress for themselves. They are not afraid to break the rules—they're their own style police.

Style Mentors know it's not about having a lot of stuff, just the right stuff.

Style Mentors know that great style is not about great cost. They feel comfortable mixing up price points when they put their look together.

Style Mentors are engaged in the adventure of life and dress for it.

Style Mentors dress to embrace who they are in the present. That's the ultimate in style. That's why they always look so great, and how you can, too.

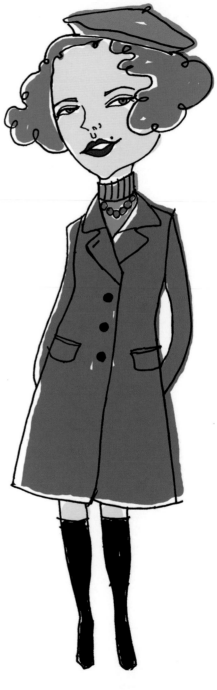

work of art

Don't limit your style wall or scrapbook to images of clothes or Style Mentors. Look to other visual sources—paintings, nature, architecture, images from travels— for inspiration.

W2W Closet Practice: Why Does She Always Look So Great?

I was an art history major in college. I'm not sure why, considering I nearly failed the subject my freshman year. I had no idea how to write an essay about a statue that had lost its arms, legs, and sometimes even the head. I stuck it out because I wanted to understand what others had been studying for centuries that I couldn't see. Eventually, I learned to appreciate the impact of light and shadow, color, gesture, proportion, focus, and storytelling. These are the same elements we employ, consciously or not, when we dress. When we get it right, we feel great. When we don't, we feel like we have flunked.

When observing Style Mentors, ask yourself:

Is it the colors she's wearing?
- Do they flatter her face and hair?
- Are they monochromatic or used as an accent?
- Do they add an element of surprise?
- Are they her part of her signature look?

Is it the way she wears her clothes?
- The fit?
- The shape?
- Do the fabrics move easily on her body, or define it?
- Do they draw attention to her assets or discreetly hide her not-so-favorite assets?
- Do they project attitude or mood?

Is it the way she puts it all together?
- Does what she is wearing appear in harmony?

Is it an accessory?
- Quirky eyeglasses, a dramatic necklace, colorful shoes, an eye-catching bag?
- Is it something she consistently wears that has become her signature piece?

Is it her hair?
- The color?
- The cut?
- The styling?

Is her makeup understated or dramatic?

Is it her body language?
- Posture?
- Gestures?
- Eye contact?
- Laugh lines?
- Does she look as if she is comfortable in what she wears?

How would you define her style?
- Classic
- Trendy
- Vintage
- Fun
- Outdoorsy
- Fashionable
- Stylish
- Hip
- Sexy
- Bohemian
- Eclectic
- Frilly
- Feminine

What do her clothes say about her?

What do my clothes say about me?

What do I want my clothes to say about me?

Ask yourself these questions when you dress.

12

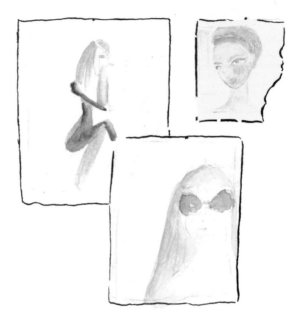

Dream a Little Dream of You

Many assume that Style Mentors possess a style gene that we don't have, just as I believed others were born with the green-thumb gene and I wasn't. Wrong. What I've found true in the garden is also true in the closet: To be pleased with the end results requires desire and focus, inspiration and information, practice and patience, and a willingness to experiment with new ideas.

Remember when you were younger and open to possibilities? You envisioned how you wanted to look on your wedding day or prom night. You thumbed through various magazines looking for ideas. You shopped and shopped trying on countless numbers of dresses until you found *the* one. When you slipped it on, you felt excited, hopeful, and pretty. You looked for flattering and attractive undergarments before making alterations so the dress would fit your body perfectly. Next was the hunt for the shoes, bag, and jewelry to complete the look.

You then looked for pictures of hairstyles to experiment with. You spent time at cosmetic counters having experts apply makeup in the way they thought complemented your face, your dress, and the occasion. Chances are you devoted the same time and attention to exercising and eating properly, so you would look and feel your best for that special occasion that would be memorialized in photographs. You succeeded! You felt connected in the very best way to what you wore and what you were experiencing in your life.

You did it then and you can do it again. By following the same steps you once did for those milestones, you can assess your body and style—and learn to look and feel great every day. With time and practice, it will become second nature.

The key elements to remember are:

Visualization is powerful—ask any successful athlete, CEO, or bride on her wedding day. When you visualize your success and repeat affirmations of your envisioned accomplishment (*I am a beautiful mother of the bride, I am a winning trial lawyer, I am a sexy wife* . . .), it can enhance your preparations to achieve your goal. The key is to visualize the positive; otherwise it will do more harm than good.

Commit to your vision. Give it time and attention until you get it right.

Be open to new possibilities. Research to find visual inspiration and then experiment by trying on new ideas. Trust your instincts as to what you like on you and what you don't.

It is about the total look, not just the dress. Make it a priority to find the right accessories and undergarments until you've got it right.

Have what you wear tailored, if necessary. Looking your best is al about fit.

Don't give up on any detail until you look great and feel fabulous.

W2W Closet Journal: The Inspiration of Imagination

When I was a fashion editor at *Town & Country* and *Esquire*, some of my responsibilities included visiting designer showrooms each season to review their collections. I was always intrigued by each designer's forever-changing wall or scrapbook compiled of images that triggered the imagination. They were often a mix of photographs from their travels, postcards, images from art books, and swatches of fabric. One collection might be a pastiche of colors, textures, and patterns found in a Moroccan bazaar, while another was influenced by the clothes worn in a Merchant-Ivory film.

By compiling your own visual style notes, you, too, will open your eyes to new possibilities of what to wear. Start by collecting images of women who have put themselves together in a manner you find appealing. Don't limit yourself to fashion magazines or pictures of celebrities. You might find images in business journals, newspapers, design and photography books, and advertisements.

By choosing images and paying attention, you will train your eye to recognize why what "she" wears works or why it doesn't. It's like watching celebrities walk the red carpet. Sometimes they look sensational; other times you wonder what they were thinking. Those who pull it off have an awareness of what looks best on them. Their clothes are an extension of their style whether on the red carpet or grocery shopping. Others are mannequins subject to trends or the whims of stylists often with costume-like results, as if they were little girls playing dress-up.

Expand your journal with other visual ideas—the way different looks are pulled together, shapes that you fancy in shoes, blouses with flourish, interesting color combinations, or new ideas on how to wear your hair. There is no right or wrong, just what pleases your eye.

As you collect images, you will start to see a theme in the styles you are drawn to. These are visual clues that will help you refine your look as you refresh your style. As your journal grows, so will your visual vocabulary. Soon you will start to feel comfortable trying on new ideas that you may not have considered otherwise.

How would you describe the overall style of the images you've placed in your style journal? These are evidence of your style preferences.

_____

_____

What are the few things in your closet that you keep replacing? These are your Closet Classics.

_____

_____

What colors do you enjoy wearing? This is your wardrobe palette.

_____

_____

Is there a consistency in what you *enjoy* wearing? This is your style signature.

_____

_____

What do you want your clothes to say about you?

_____

_____

How would you define your style?

_____

_____

Closet Confidential: *Style Confidence*

"I used to dress to fit in when I was a young woman; now I dress to stand out. I often mix very expensive clothes or jewelry with inexpensive pieces that I may have bought off the street. It's the way you layer things, and how you put them together in your own creative way, which depends on the emotions of the day. There is no right or wrong, there is just pretty and ugly. My signature piece is a large Chanel cross on a heavy chain. It's bold and attractive and I love to wear it!"

Carmen, seventy-seven, world-famous model

"When I was in college, I was borderline hippie. I wore a long braid to my waist, lots of Marimekko prints and torn-looking clothes from South America. I still harbor a fantasy of costumes, especially when I have to wear dressy clothes. I would rather wear brocades and vintage flapper dresses than the perfect black dress. The dropped waist flatters my figure. They have become one of my trademarks for dressy occasions. During the day I absolutely cannot live without black pants, a black sweater, black T-shirt, and a little black dress. Those staples have been consistent throughout my life. I wear the clothes I love over and over again."

Ellen, sixty, magazine executive, Manhattan

"My style is consistent—classic preppy with a twist: fun tights, a ruffle or tuxedo shirt, and belts. Jewelry can change an outfit dramatically. My clothes are basically black, white, and cream. I add color with long Loro Piana scarves—they are my signature pieces. And I love jeans, especially my Levi's. The way I dress says a lot about me—that I'm sporty, confident, and somewhat private. I don't want to show everything upfront so I stay away from anything low-cut or revealing. And my shoes indicate my moods."

Kathy, forty-five, interior designer, San Francisco

I was inspired by a woman dressed in black with a large turquoise wrap worn tossed over one shoulder. She radiated style. Another woman draped hers around her shoulders, the long end thrown back over a shoulder in a dramatic sweep that was functional, glamorous, and forgiving of body bulges.

unexpected

If your wardrobe is in the doldrums,
give it a lift by adding one unexpected item to the mix. It can be as
eye-catching as a decorative coat, or
as subtle as the flounce of a jacket.
The idea is that it expresses how you
want to *feel* in your clothes.

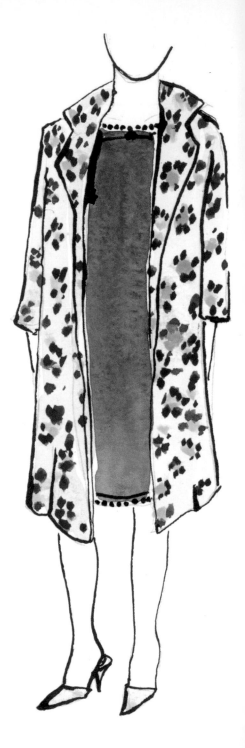

"It's dispiriting when women of a certain age sink into wearing all-beige or other bland colors. They look like melting candles. I like wearing color—aqua, yellow, orange, green, and I love red. It cheers me up! I also make an effort to achieve balance by calmly, not frantically, trying new things, and not rejecting the old just because they're old. I may be old myself, but I don't want to be stuck in the past. It's a fine line to walk. My closet standbys are bangles, vintage faux jewelry, and a wide gold chain watch—I've replaced the face with pictures of my grandchildren. I like wearing stretch velvet jeans, black pants, long-sleeved jewel-neck sweaters, and a particular favorite is a sweater jacket with fox trim that I can throw over most everything I wear."

Diane, sixty-four, design writer, Manhattan

"My daughter tells me that my style is more glamorous now than when I was younger. I think it's because I try harder. As we age, all women should pay more attention to their style."

Kathryn, sixty-five, writer, Manhattan

I define my style as simple basics in black and white with a twist: a decorative coat, a flourish of ruffles, animal prints, textured hosiery, leather skirts. Large jewelry is important to me, in part because it helps to draw the eye away from my larger middle, but also because it's festive. My signature pieces are a large black wooden ring, gold hoop earrings, and an oversize heart-shaped crystal by jewelry designer Kazuko that dangles on a cord that I wear around my neck. I've noticed how my style journal (those photos that I tape on the inside of my closet door) is crowded with images of increasingly bolder design gestures.

Now I need to figure out what style of classics and twists will best suit my changing body.

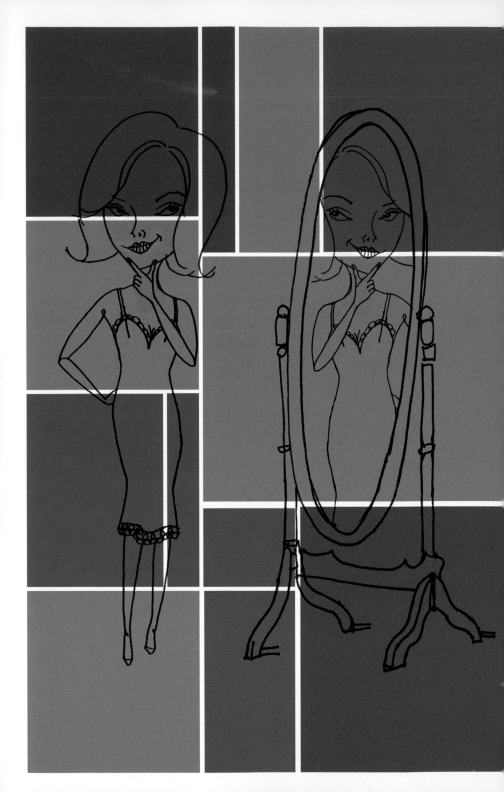

Don't try to
be original.
Just try to
be good.
—Paul Rand

PART THREE
HOW DO I LOOK?

When I see
a woman I
don't see
what's wrong
with her, I see
what's right.
—Bobbi Brown

13

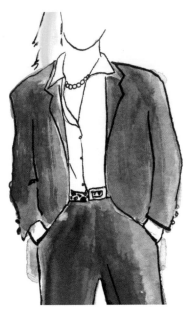

Evolving Closets

I recently found a photograph that was taken of me several years ago for a Japanese magazine. It was taken in the Soho, New York, office where I worked for many years on the Chic Simple books. I look confident standing tall in my ankle-high, zip-front black suede snow boots designed by a very fancy French designer. My straight shoulder-length hair was blunt-cut and sun-bleached rather than softly layered and artificially brightened as it is today. My body appears trim, dressed in the well-cut black cashmere blazer I bought when covering the Italian fashion collections for *Esquire* magazine in days when the dollar was mighty and my paycheck was steady. I had tucked my crisp white cotton tailored shirt into skinny black jeans that were fastened at the waist by a thin leopard-print belt, which added a splash of dash to my dependable basics.

I enjoyed wearing these functional, efficient clothes for a memorable stretch of time in my life. They were my work uniform in the office and on book tours to Australia, Japan, London, and the northern cities across the United States—they looked too city-slick and somber for the pretty, colorful clothing cultures of Atlanta, Texas, and Southern California. I wore these clothes as mom—accompanying my children's elementary school class on outings to museums, nature preserves, and the Statue of Liberty; as an art docent; and attending the school plays, dance recitals, and athletic events they participated in. They were the clothes I threw on to rush to the emergency room after I got the call that my mother had been in a serious car accident, and when I accompanied her to doctor appointments once she was diagnosed with cancer.

I can't remember when these indispensable favorites disappeared from my closet. The jeans had stretch, but not enough as my middle gradually filled out over the years. I wore the jacket the way a young child wears a security blanket. After much use, it grew threadbare and became part of my weekend uniform—until one day its broad shoulders also betrayed its age. The classic white shirt, which *might* still fit, has vanished. I suspect it was left behind in my marriage, likely mixed up with those that belonged to my ex-husband, and long forgotten by each of us. I still wear the boots, but I'm not even vaguely aware of when I stopped wearing this favorite belt—or any belt for that matter.

Except for the telltale size of the jacket's shoulders, these clothes were classics. They survived the years in style, but my body had changed. We may feel young and strong, yet despite healthy diets and fitness regimens, for many of us our weight has shifted as our hormones have changed. Even if we still fit into the clothes we have worn for years, they may not be as flattering as they used to be.

The black turtlenecks I once counted on for style cool and body warmth now accentuate my jowls (a junior Alien in the making), which I otherwise choose not to notice. My legs remain shapely, but with age have become uneven in color. I no longer cavalierly parade bare-legged. It's now a thoughtful decision on hot summer days made after slathering on self-tanner. Besides, the short skirts I once wore now feel appropriate only on the beach. And because of my burgeoning middle, there is no way I can wear anything tucked in or belted at the waist.

One morning we wake up, lazily glance in the mirror, and can't quite believe that the turkey chin that gave our dad's face "character" has roosted on our once clean jawline. We've already noticed how our mother's Buddha belly thinks it's found harmony within us, too. And ouch! Those stilettos that gave us a sexy lift are at war with our bunions and self-image. We're growing into our genes and unfortunately our jeans no longer fit.

Whether it's a weight gain, weight shift, thinning hair, or our body's now insistent demand for physical comfort, as our bodies evolve, so must our wardrobe. While we may not be able to control the spread of our girth, we can control what we wear to look and feel our best.

Our closets don't need an overhaul every time our bodies undergo change. It's an evolution, not a revolution. It requires awareness as to how we can wear our clothes in a better way to suit our changing bodies, and being open to new style possibilities when replacing our outgrown or worn-out basics. Our bodies can look entirely different depending on what we wear and how we wear it. When I look at this picture, I am reminded that while the items have changed, the style remains—I just need to wear it all differently today.

14

How to Wear a Shirt When You No Longer Have a Waist and Other Closet Dramas

I said the word "vagina" "vagina" "vagina" a million times. I thought I was home free. I had finally come to like my vagina. Until one day I realized the self-hatred had just crept up into my stomach . . . It has protruded through my clothes, my confidence and my ability to work. —Eve Ensler, *The Good Body*

We know we're in closet confusion when our clothes make us feel bad about our bodies and ourselves. Simply put, as our bodies change, so must what we wear and how we wear it. When we wear clothes that fit and feel comfortable, we feel better about our bodies and ourselves. With the right-fitting pants, even Eve Ensler might grow to like—okay, accept—her stomach as much as her vagina.

Let's hear it again, gals: *When you are clothes-confident you will feel more body-confident, which will help you feel life-confident.*

This doesn't mean that the more clothes you have or the more expensive they are, the more confident you will be. It means that when you *feel* good in your clothes, you will feel better about your body and more confident dealing with the rest of your life.

Having had a long career as a fashion editor and author, I am aware of the many edicts my colleagues and I have put forth over the years telling women how to dress their best. There is much conflicting advice, because each of us writes from our personal perspective at a particular moment in our own lives to a diverse audience varying in age, body type, lifestyle, preferences, and budget. The bottom line is to know the rules then break them as you wish, or at least after experimenting. And be your own judge. You'll know you've got it right when you can smile when wearing your clothes, rather than feeling tormented.

Style Rules That Never Change

DISTRACT BY ATTRACTING. Strategically draw attention to an asset or away from a not-so-very-favorite asset. I often wear a bold necklace and patterned hosiery so the eye is drawn to my face and to my legs and away from my protruding middle.

ACHIEVE VISUAL BALANCE. When you hear the word *proportion* in terms of clothes, think balance. For example, a wide-open neckline will play up your shoulders and counterbalance wide hips or thighs. Balance voluminous pants with fitted tops, and roomy tops with fitted bottoms. In general, when putting an outfit together, opposites attract—except when it comes to shoes and hair. Delicate shoes look best with delicate clothes. Chunkier shoes look better with chunkier clothes (that doesn't sound very pretty, but you get the idea). Long hair suits a long neck, short hair flatters a short neck.

FIT IS CRITICAL TO LOOKING YOUR BEST. If what you wear is tight, you'll feel fat. If it's baggy, you'll look fat. If it fits, you will feel comfortable and look great. Fabrics with a bit of stretch are our new best friends. If your clothes need a nip and tuck for shape, find a good tailor. Add the service into your wardrobe budget before you shop.

DON'T FOLLOW FASHION TRENDS. WEAR WHAT LOOKS GOOD ON YOUR BODY. Those are the clothes that will become your Closet Classics and should be at arm's reach in your Feel-Good Closet.

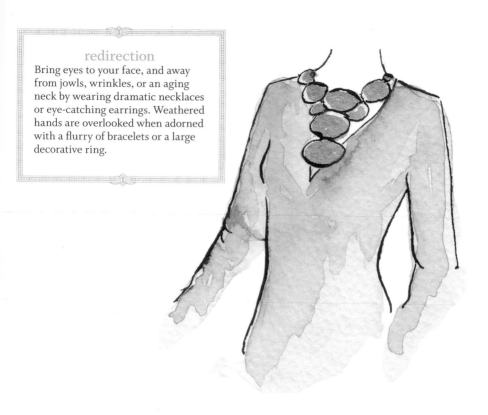
USE COLOR TO YOUR ADVANTAGE. Everyone's body looks best wearing a base of neutral monochromatic tones for a clean, slimming, and elongated line. The darker the color, the thinner you will appear. Neutrals also make it easier to update your look by adding a splash of color or a pattern, or highlight an accessory. Choosing a color palette for your wardrobe will make it easier to mix and match your clothes. A flattering color placed near your face will give it a youthful glow. The wrong color will make you appear drawn.

PAY ATTENTION! The one thing you can count on in life is change. Use the mirror as an analytical tool and be in touch with your body and your Feel-Good Closet. Never give up on your closet or yourself!

Mirror Talk: Managing Your Assets

I love myself, I really do, except when I have to get dressed.
—Ali, thirty-nine, Feng Shui consultant, Brooklyn, New York

If you think you look better naked than when you are wearing clothes, you are not dressing your best. The how-to-dress for your body rules haven't changed, but our bodies have. We need to become acquainted with our new body and reacquainted with the rules that now apply to us.

Look in the mirror with an uncritical eye. Acknowledge what you like about your body now. Assets don't vanish with time; they merely change. We all have at least a few. *Revisit the assets you recorded earlier in your W2W Closet Journal.* You'll become more cognizant of dressing them up.

Next, write down what you consider your most annoying body issues—prioritize. Again, don't be critical, just analytical.

When you get into your closet, start by dressing the most challenging part of your body, or conversely with something that flatters your best feature. Then be mindful of the balancing act as you add other pieces of clothing and accessories.

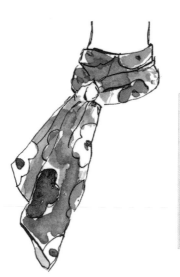

Closet Confidential: Balancing Act

"When I get dressed, I try to take time and experiment to see what works
best with what. I think about what fabrics look best together, and if it's
'hanging right.' Then I think about what kind of accessory would make
the outfit. The necklace and earrings I choose often indicate the season
by their color and style."

Goldie, sixty-three, health care administrative assistant,
Yonkers, New York

"Sometimes I put an outfit together around a pair of shoes or a
decorative scarf or a patterned skirt. It's always about the mood."

Beatriz, forty-nine, CEO of HispanAmérica and
power yoga teacher, Newfoundland, Pennsylvania

Dress for Your Neck

If you have an aging neck, hiding it in a turtleneck is not necessarily the
best solution. It's not always practical, comfortable, or flattering, especially
if you have a short neck, full face, or jowls, or you suffer hot flashes. A
cowl neck or a colorful scarf looped around the neck is a softer alternative.
Or distract by attracting—wear a dazzling necklace (faux is fabulous), an

upturned shirt collar in a flattering color, or short decorative earrings. Play up your hair and your eyewear. Each of these elements will beautifully frame your face rather than draw attention down to your neck.

If you have a long neck, turtlenecks, cowl necks, mandarin collars, a high but horizontally opened neckline (boat neck, bateau, Sabrina), turned-up collars, multistranded chokers, long dramatic earrings, shoulder-length hair, and bangs (if your chin is clean and your face not overly round) all bring balance to a long neck.

If you have a short neck, avoid chokers, turtlenecks, and jewel necklines. Create vertical length with open collars, deep V-necks, wide scoop necks, and off-the-shoulder necklines. Keep hair short and off the neck. Long earrings are great for short necks because they give the illusion of length and bring the eye upward.

Dress for Your Shoulders

Shoulders (and legs) are the slowest parts of your body to show their age—and they're sexy! Everyone looks great with a degree of an open, horizontal neckline. Baring shoulders, even a bit, balances wide hips, thighs, and a thick midriff. Play them up!

If your shoulders are broad, stay away from shoulder pads and avoid wearing oversized sleeves, jewel necklines, off-the-shoulder necklines, and ballerina necklines (a wide shallow scoop). They all make shoulders appear wider. Halter tops with deep armholes, and strapless tops will flatter.

Conversely, **if you have narrow shoulders,** do the opposite, but replace any football-size shoulder pads, which look dated, with a softer, subtler version.

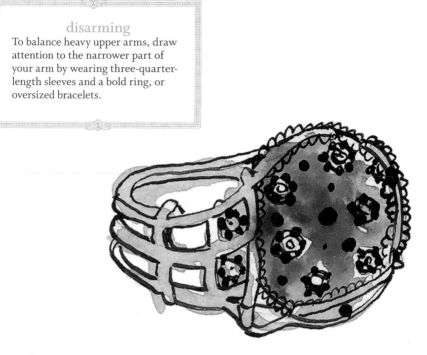
Dress for Your Arms

To bare or not to bare the upper arms is a personal comfort call. If you are on the fence, wraps or sheer cover-ups are great solutions when dressing up.

If your upper arms have grown heavy, wear sleeves but accentuate your shoulders with a wide, soft ballerina scoop neck and off-the-shoulder tops. Stay away from cap sleeves. V-necks and turned-up collars also bring focus away from upper arms. Elbow-length and three-quarter-length bracelet sleeves are stylish (look at first ladies Jackie O and Michelle O) and flattering because they balance the upper arm by revealing a slender part of your arm. Exaggerated sleeves or those that flare at the wrist in a delicate, blousy fabric are also a great counterbalance to heavy upper arms. Medium to small-size prints are a festive distraction. Wearing bold jewelry at your wrist, a large cocktail ring, or a substantial necklace also draws the eye away from upper arms.

Dress for Your Cleavage

When I was in my early forties, I needed an evening dress for several black-tie events. I bought a fabulous black one by Donna Karan that was long in the back and cut short in the front, which showed off my legs. It had a low scoop stretch velvet neckline, which required me to buy a new bra. I found a strapless one that commandeered everything I had up, out, and together. It was the very first time in my life that men talked to me while looking at my cleavage. Those who knew me actually blushed. I loved it! I had a glimpse of the sexual power that women with cleavage know. It felt great to be part of the cognoscenti. It was all about what I was wearing, not about the reality of what was underneath. I wasn't on the prowl and soon to be found out, so I could simply relish the feeling. It felt like womanly fun.

If your cleavage is no longer holding up, buy a bra that lifts. Make an appointment with an expert fitter in a lingerie department or specialty store to make sure you are still wearing the correct size. A bra that fits properly will help your body appear younger and trimmer.

If you have petite breasts, chances are they have increased in size since menopause or weight gain. Getting refitted for a bra will show your breasts off at their best. Some bras will push everything you have up and give you *wow* cleavage. (Industry secret of sorts: Professional stylists often tape celebrities' breasts up and together for the illusion of cleavage.)

Tops with a decorative flourish in front—cascading ruffles, shirring—give the illusion of breasts, by obscuring their size.

Other ways to flatter **petite breasts** are by wearing halter necks or off-the-shoulder tops. Jewel and bateau necklines (look to Audrey Hepburn) will help your breasts appear larger. Bulky knits and turtlenecks also flatter my petite-bosomed comrades, but we should stay away from empire necklines—they work better for our **large-breasted** sisters.

Wrap tops and dresses flatter both **large and small breasts,** because they give the illusion of a waist, which creates balance. Fabrics should caress your breasts. Too-tight or too-loose tops are unflattering. Stretchy fabrics will give you a better fit.

If you are large-breasted, stay away from boxy or double-breasted jackets. They will make you look, well, boxy. Fitted jackets with a deep V and small lapels will flatter. A control camisole under a wrap top will help to keep everything in place. Be sure it's cut high and has wide shoulder straps to hide your bra minimizer.

Avoid excess detailing near your breasts—pockets, wide lapels, and ruffles—and beware of long necklaces that cascade off your chest. Bulky knits will make you look—you got it—bulky. Scoop and jewel necklines make large breasts appear even larger. Shirring under the bust will diminish large breasts. Strapless tops, V-necks, and sweetheart necklines also look great.

If you're having trouble fitting into a shirt, buy it larger and have darts or seams inserted by a tailor to softly shape it under your bustline. It will also give the illusion of a smaller waistline. If you are of average height and short-waisted, you may have better luck finding shirts that fit in the petite department.

A belted waist will make you appear top-heavy, but a fitted waist with a full skirt and an open neckline will create an attractive uplifting silhouette. Skinny pants and narrow skirts will also make you appear top-heavy. A-line or softly draped skirts and dresses, as well as full pants and those that flare, will all flatter because they will counterbalance large breasts. Wearing darker colors on top will visually diminish large breasts, especially when wearing brighter colors or patterns below for balance.

If your décolletage is wrinkled or sun-damaged, wear a peakaboo mesh top or one in a semi-sheer fabric to obscure it. Diane, a sixty-four-year-old design writer, considers Sophia Loren the Queen of Mesh. "It's sexy and it holds everything in." Fashion designer Kay Unger recommends wearing piles and piles of necklaces on a bare décolletage—"It's sexy whatever your age!"

If you decide to wear a high neckline, reveal some of your back, shoulders, or arms. And think about showing off your legs if they are fetching. Legs can be as sexy as décolletage.

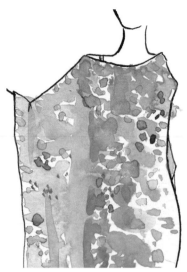

Dress for Your Back

Coco Chanel hated women's knees, so when she designed evening wear she emphasized a woman's back. Fast-forward to Hollywood in 2005 when Hilary Swank picked up her Best Actress Oscar wearing what appeared to be a chaste-looking long-sleeved, high-neck fitted dress . . . until she turned her back to the camera to reveal a provocatively low-cut back.

A drop back or cutout keyhole back is alluring, and sometimes referred to as rear cleavage—an appealing alternative when things aren't going well with our décolletage or frontal cleavage. It also brings attention to the derriere.

Bras are available to accommodate a drop back, but let's get real. Many of us have back flab now that is not sexy, so be mindful of how much back you reveal. Back rolls are more visible when you're wearing the wrong-size bra or anything else on top that's tight or clingy.

BAG BACKS

A few years ago, I was at a gathering where a superstar magician performed parlor magic and clairvoyance readings. He told a random woman from the audience that she had a pain in her knee. She did. Actually I did, too. He later clued us in that a high percentage of women suffer knee problems because most of us carry heavy bags. This throws our alignment off, impacting the knees.

Bags add color, panache, and personality to what we wear, but for many of us, they have become mini suitcases that we park on our shoulders. If you need to schlep lots of stuff, choose bags that are lightweight or that distribute your weight evenly on both shoulders.

For visual balance, your bag should be proportionate to your body. If you are petite, a big purse will dwarf you. If you have a large build, a small purse will in contrast emphasize your size. If you have large breasts, wear the bag lower on your body to draw the eye down. If your hips or thighs are wide, wear the bag higher up on your shoulder to bring the eye upward. The dressier the occasion, the smaller the bag should be.

Dress for Your Waist

If you have a trim waist, show it off with fitted (not tight) tops, belted jackets, and wrap dresses. Pants with contour waistbands are flattering especially for women with small waists and curvy hips.

For us thick-waisted gals, a body shaper will manage your midriff. If your middle is thicker than your bust, wear a padded push-up bra for balance.

Pants that are full-cut, straight-legged from the hip, or boot-cut counter balance a thick middle. Don't even think about tucking in tops or wearing belts at the waist. Belts that sit on your hip are more flattering.

Stay away from pockets in the front unless they're jeans (you can always cut out the inner pockets and sew them up to rid yourself of extra fabric). If you find great-fitting pants with belt loops, remove the loops.

Pull-on pants are an easy fit. Don't screech! They are great, great, great (and comfortable), but *only* if the waistband lies flat so that it doesn't add bulkiness. They look even better when they are cut with hidden seams for contour. Never tuck in your top.

Pleated skirts need to be stitched down to mid-hip to avoid fullness around the waist, stomach, and hips. Slim-cut skirts, especially those with a flounce, are a great option.

When flab protrudes above your waistband, aka **muffin top,** it means you are wearing the wrong size or a style not suited for your body. A tailor can usually let out a waistband.

the wrap

Since 1972, when Diane von Furstenberg created the wrap dress, it's been a Closet Classic. The flattering cut enhances the bust and trims the waist. The deep V-neck elongates the body, which brings the eye upward. Busy prints can camouflage. And it's as versatile as your closet. It looks hip worn with boots and a statement belt, or elegant with sensible pumps and a string of pearls.

If your waist is thick or you are short-waisted, stay away from shirtwaist dresses. Shift dresses and sheaths are attractive alternatives. Dresses that skim the waist and stomach and that are slightly fuller at the bottom are flattering, as are those with a dropped waist.

For the illusion of a waist, off-the-shoulder tops will make your waist appear smaller. Wrap dresses can also flatter. The deep V-neck brings the eye upward to provide a long, graceful line.

Tailored jackets give shape to your waist, especially when narrowly cut or cinched at the waist. A peplum also creates a great silhouette. If you find a few in your closet but can no longer button them, wear them unbuttoned (fake it!).

Fabrics should skim, not hug, your middle. A blouse with a decorative element in front, like a flourish of ruffles or ruching, detracts the eye from the waist. Rib knits stitched strategically can be slimming and give the illusion of a smaller waistline.

Use accessories to bring the eye upward—a long colorful looped scarf, a piece of big jewelry worn from the chest up, dramatic glasses.

So very sad for us thick- and short-waisted gals, but the classic, glorious, mysterious trench coat doesn't work unless the trench is cut in a stiff fabric so it flares from the waist.

Dress for Your Stomach

Closet Confidential: *Body Style*

"I am high-waisted and have a little tummy. To downplay my tummy, I wear narrow skirts and will only wear a pleated skirt if the pleats are sewn down to below my tummy. I also like narrow pants and stay away from those with pleats. I don't think pleats camouflage the stomach. I like a princess line to elongate my waist, and I wear belts that lie on my hips. I have hippie belts from the 1960s with grommets that I still wear. I like a softer silhouette on top. I love Anne Fontaine shirts. They have a tailored bottom so you don't have to tuck them in."

Ellen, sixty, magazine executive, Manhattan

When your stomach isn't flat, tops look best worn untucked (wear those that are hemmed for a neat look) and resting comfortably mid-tummy. As your stomach and middle expand, the tops you have had over the years creep up in length, which will emphasize your stomach.

Balance a swollen tummy by wearing a push-up padded bra, dramatic sleeves that billow, open necklines, and tops with shirring or ruffles that flourish above the stomach.

A thin part of your torso is the area just below your bust. Dresses with raised waistlines or those that are fitted at the breasts and then slightly flare are flattering, as are empire silhouettes.

Fabric with some weight will give you better shape. Beware of lightweight fabrics or your stomach might look voluminous.

Dress-and-jacket combinations look pulled together and diminish a thick middle.

A tailored jacket with shape or a bit of peplum will detract from the stomach.

Vests are my new favorites, especially for casual dressing. They can add an interesting color or texture (Polarfleece, leather . . .), especially when worn over a solid column of neutral color. They're also heaven-sent for fluctuating body temperatures, are easy to move in, and cover up a thick or lumpy middle.

Use color and bold accessories to attract the eye away from your stomach.

To avoid extra bulk, remove the inside fabric of pants pockets and stitch the pockets closed. Stay away from front zippers and waistbands that don't lie flat or are tight. Waistbands should lie just below the waist. Choose flat front pants over pleats.

If you're wearing an empire cut, be sure that the fabric isn't so voluminous that it makes you look pregnant. I have a photograph of supermodel Gisele Bundchen looking positively pregnant because the dress she was wearing had too much fabric cascading from beneath her chest.

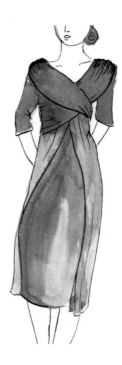

Dress for Your Hips and Thighs

Closet Confidential: Hip Hips

"Wearing a column of a solid color such as black, beige, navy, et cetera, is good under a jacket worn open or closed. If you have full hips, the column should be dark."

Nina McLemore, fashion designer, Manhattan

If you have large hips, avoid baggy tees and long tops, which will appear tent-like. Long jackets and shirts will make you look wider and shorter. Tops should end at the hip. Balance with a wide or off-the-shoulder neckline, or a blousy shirt with dramatic sleeves. Jazz up the bodice and keep everything below the waist simple to bring the eye upward.

Jackets with bold lapels balance full hips. Fitted jackets that flare below the waist also diminish broad hips. Wear color above the waist to attract the eye upward, and dark monochromatic tones below to diminish size.

Pants should sit at the top of the hip. Don't wear belts at your waist. Remove belt loops.

Pants that have a narrow leg or that taper at the hem will emphasize hips. Stay away from pleats—they'll likely pull. Horizontal pockets and vertical side pockets in the side seam of pants will make you look broader. Diagonal pockets are more flattering.

Lined pants will help conceal cellulite.

Stay away from bias-cut or pencil skirts. A-line skirts skim over hips, making them appear smaller.

> Bias-cutting is a technique used by designers for cutting clothing in the diagonal direction of a fabric so it drapes softly on the body, accentuating curves. The technique is used most frequently for dresses, but in the Middle Ages, before knitting, hose was cut on the bias for a better fit.

Tops with a wide round neckline worn with a slightly flared skirt or pants that are full-legged will soften the line of your hips.

If you have a flat stomach and wide hips or thighs, wear a tailored dress in a stiff fabric, like satin or wool, with a princess silhouette. Or look for one with a raised waist that gradually flares out, skimming your hips and thighs. These shapes will accentuate your waist and your bustline, while diminishing your hips.

Dress for Your Derriere

Closet Confidential: *Shapely Solution*

"I've always had a lousy ass, so I downplay it. I have a great bias-cut dress by Jackie Rogers—a bias cut is very flattering to the body."

Carmen, seventy-seven, world-famous model

If you are losing your butt or developing secretary's spread, find the right body shaper to give you a lift or pull you in. Wearing heels also gives the derriere a boost.

Have pencil skirts and fitted dresses tailored to give some shape to your behind.

Skirts with black pleats or a rear flounce are feminine and flirty.

To diminish your butt, wear skirts in heavy fabrics that provide shape.

Don't emphasize your small waist.

Jackets should be fitted and flare out from the waist or skim your butt while covering it.

Balance a large derriere with pants that sit below your waist and that are boot-cut or wide-legged. Tapered trousers are a no-no.

Avoid rear pockets, but if they're a necessity, they should be large. Small ones will only make your butt appear bigger. No pleats.

Fabrics that are tightly woven give support and those with a bit of stretch provide shape.

If your derriere is disappearing, look for skirts with rear pleats or pockets, a flounce, or a rear seam that can be easily altered for more definition.

The rise in a pant is the distance between the crotch seam and the top of the waist. If your pants are baggy in the crotch, you need a shorter rise. If pants or skirts fit your derriere but not your waist, have the waistband tailored.

Lower-cut pants look good on me because I have a flat bum, even if they're meant for younger girls. I like the contemporary styles, but do however feel they should not be skintight on women of a certain age.
—gg, forty-plus, cosmetics entrepreneur, Rockport, Maine

Dress for Your Legs

Legs are slow to lose their shape. The best skirt length hovers around the knee. Wear it slightly above if your legs are great, or just below if your knees aren't. And you can't go wrong with a mid-knee hem. It's classic.

If you want a long-legged look, try a slim-fitting pant with a slightly flared leg (boot cut) or full-cut pants, and wear heels. Hosiery should be a similar color to pants or shoes so the vertical line isn't broken. Or wear a black skirt with black tights and black boots for a long, lean, leggy look.

If you have shapely legs, but they have become mottled over the years with brown sun spots or visible or unsightly veins, deciding to bare them or not is much like deciding whether to bare your arms.

There are varieties of cosmetic options to correct these nuisances, but for the majority of us, it's way down on our to-do list.

For summer legs, many of us opt for a self-tanner. (My favorite is Jergens Natural Glow Express Daily Moisturizer, which I often mix with a body moisturizer before applying for a smooth finish.) Nude fishnet hosiery is a hip and sexy alternative. And you can't go wrong with those in sheer nude or black. Stay away from white unless you work in a hospital.

For cool weather, opaque tights and patterned hosiery will stylishly play up your legs.

If you have thick ankles, pants should be long enough to hide them. But wear a fun or sexy shoe for diversion (not one with straps, though). For balance, wear skirts that hover around the knee and have a slight flare.

Dress for Your Feet

LOVE YOUR FEET!

I attended a seminar at my alma mater honoring the 150 years since women were first admitted to what was originally a men's university. I was surprised to see several women who were leaders in a variety of industries—medicine, broadcasting, finance, beauty, politics—seated on stage for a symposium wearing kick-ass high heels. I thought, *Wow, we've come a long way, baby, but at what price?* High heels communicate sex and power, but ouch!

Shoes are the quickest way to change the personality of what we wear. Think jeans worn with clogs, boots, heels, sneakers—you get the idea.

They help us perform better, create a mood, and—much like a sadomasochistic dominatrix—can hold our body in bondage. Sound sexy? Well, for some it might be, but for many of us it's not, and the results can be ugly.

I love walking and I love shoes. When I was in my early forties, I woke up to step into a nightmare of excruciating pain that throbbed in the ball of my foot. Clueless, I hobbled to an orthopedic doctor, who diagnosed that I had worn down the fat padding that cushions the feet—their shock absorbers. The culprits were the flip-flops, espadrilles, and other loose fitting, nonsupportive shoes I had been running around in far too long.

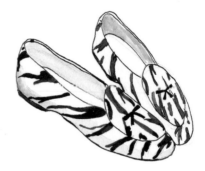

comfort chic
Belgian shoes are the grown-up version of the Pappagallos we wore in the sixties, but they're exceptionally comfortable (and they're available!). The hand-stitched slippers come in animal prints and a rainbow of color combinations. Be sure to have soles applied. www.belgianshoes.com

Morton's neuroma is a nerve inflammation that results in a severe burning pain on the ball of the foot, often a result of wearing very tight or very unstructured shoes. Orthotics, anti-inflammatory drugs, and padded shoes help to alleviate the symptoms.

I had orthopedic inserts made for my sneakers and began my collection of Belgian shoes—which fashion pros and aging WASPS, male and female, know are extraordinarily comfortable and the epitome of classic chic (my favorites are the animal prints). I then searched for a pair of dressy shoes that I could wear to important meetings and special events without aggravating my condition. I was thrilled that I could justify buying a pair of pricey Manolo Blahnik kitten heels. I've been wearing them comfortably and stylishly for more than a decade. Talk about investment dressing! My summer weekend shoes of choice were, and remain, clogs and Birkenstocks. Don't cringe. Even model-*cum*-designer Heidi Klum designs her own line of hip Birkenstock footwear, and every spring there is a deluge of designer rip-offs in fashionable colors. Why? Because our feet hurt! Apparently by age forty, approximately 80 percent of us have some sort of foot or ankle problem, and between the ages of fifty and fifty-five that number increases to 90 percent.

I joyfully wear these shoes. To me comfort is the new chic.

Most podiatrists agree that heels higher than two inches are too high. It's silly to see women teetering painfully in stilettos. It's equally unattractive to wear athletic shoes for anything other than sports, especially now that the footwear industry has been developing stylish shoes with orthopedic ergonomics and athletic support technology.

Simply put, don't wear high heels that hurt. If they do, it's because your body is trying to tell you something. If you can't help yourself, don't stand in them for more than an hour and don't walk in them more than a block. Also, insert gel pads to absorb some of the shock.

Closet Confidential: Heeling Closet

"Shoes can influence how you move and feel as a woman. I can't run around in heels anymore. The older I get, the lower the heel. If your feet are uncomfortable, I don't think you can be happy. Your feet get more sensitive with age. If I'm wearing a heel, I'll insert a gel pad for the ball of my foot. At night when I put on my sweatpants, a very soft top, and Pumas with the Velcro strap, my body immediately relaxes."

Dayle Haddon, fifty-five, UNICEF ambassador,
L'Oréal spokesperson, and best-selling author

The plantar fascia is a shock absorber that supports the arch in your feet. Stress overload (bearing heavy weight or participating in sports that pound the feet) can leave you with small tears in the fascia, resulting in excruciating heel pain. It is usually felt first thing in the morning when your muscles have contracted overnight, or after long periods of standing or sitting. The best shoes to wear for this condition are those with a low to moderate heel, good arch support, and shock absorbency.

THE WORST SHOES YOU CAN WEAR

- Shoes that have thin or stiff soles or lack arch support don't provide the shock support needed to protect your feet, knees, and back. When the stress becomes too great, it can result in plantar fasciitis—an incredible pain in your heels.
- Shoes that are unstructured or too tight can cause nerve inflammation that manifests as a burning pain on the balls of your feet.
- Shoes so loose that you must grip your toes to keep them on can cause small tears in the ligaments of your foot.
- Inflexible shoe soles are a common cause of shin splints.
- Shoes that are tight and squish your toes can also cause or aggravate bunions, hammer toes, and corns.
- High-heel addicts are contracting their Achilles' tendon, which strains the tissue around the heel and can cause muscle spasms. High heels also put a huge amount of stress on the ball of the foot, which can cause a stress fracture.
- Don't wear worn-out athletic shoes. They lose cushion and support with use.

***Closet Confidential:* Comfort Chic**

"I don't need a lot of shoes, but I need comfortable ones. And because of my bunions, I wear flats. I like Stubbs & Wootton decorative needlepoint shoes, because they breathe and stretch without being so soft to reveal the ugly shape of my feet."

Julia, fifty-plus, art consultant, Richfield, Idaho

THE BEST SHOES YOU CAN WEAR

- **If you have short calf muscles,** they will feel better in a slight heel. Low heels also prevent muscles from becoming overstretched, and will help your legs appear longer than they would in flats.
- Thick heels, wedges, and platform shoes distribute body weight more evenly than narrow heels, which is easier on our skeletons.
- **If you have high arches,** they need cushioning.
- **If you have flat feet,** they need arch support.

- Shoes with pointy toes may be stylish, but will hurt your feet if your toes are uncomfortable.
- **Alternate the shoes you wear as often as possible.**

SHOP SMART FOR SHOES

Closet Confidential: Get Real

"I buy reality, not fantasy. I have foot problems. If you can't walk, you can't think. When your body is out of kilter, it affects your mind. I like Taryn Rose shoes. They feel good on my feet."

Carmen, seventy-seven, world-famous model

Never assume you know your size. Feet expand with weight gain, during pregnancy, when you are physically active, and with age. And as with clothes, sizing varies among manufacturers.

Shoes should be comfortable when you buy them. Never buy shoes that are tight with the intent of breaking them in. They will aggravate corns and bunions.

Buy shoes late in the day when your feet are most swollen. That being said, don't wear brand-new shoes for a special occasion without a trial run.

My mother was in a car accident that damaged one of her feet. Arthritis set in, causing one foot to become larger than the other. What to do? Some stores offer split pairs of shoes or discounts on the second pair purchased. Nordstrom sells mismatched pairs without a surcharge to people whose feet differ by at least a size and a half. If you buy two different sizes, consider donating the unworn mismatched shoes to the National Odd Shoe Exchange (www.oddshoe.org), a nonprofit group that provides new shoes to amputees and to people with significantly mismatched feet. Birkenstock Express, the mail-order service of Footwise Inc. based in Corvallis, Oregon, will sell individual shoes in select styles or discount second pairs. Custom-made footwear is a pricey alternative.

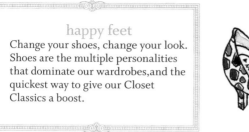
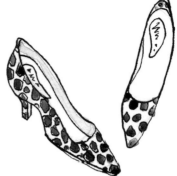

> ### happy feet
> Change your shoes, change your look.
> Shoes are the multiple personalities
> that dominate our wardrobes, and the
> quickest way to give our Closet
> Classics a boost.

Closet Confidential: *I Am Wear I Am*

"There is totally completely a connection to mood and the clothes you wear.
In the morning you should think about where am I going, what am I doing
and what do I want to project. If you're active, running around you want
good, practical shoes. If you are having a flirty lunch, put on the heels."

Diane von Furstenberg, fashion designer

**When it comes to choosing shoes to wear with your clothes, opposites don't
attract.** When your clothes are heavy or bulky looking, they require a
sturdy-looking shoe. Delicate outfits need delicate shoes. The beefier the
hosiery, the more solid looking the shoe. The sheerer the hosiery, the more
delicate the shoe. The shorter the hem (pants and skirts), the shorter the
heel. Dark clothes look better with dark shoes; light clothes look better
with light-colored shoes.

**Capri pants look best with flats and mules. Skinny jeans look great with flats.
Wide-legged pants look best with heels or chunky shoes.** With long pants,
there should be no gap between the hem and the top of your shoes. Socks
should be high enough so there is no skin exposure when you sit.

To elongate the look of your leg, match the color of your shoes with your
hosiery, skirt, or pants. The darker they are, the longer and slimmer your

legs will appear. This trick will also diminish large feet and thick ankles. **If you prefer nude-colored hosiery when wearing skirts and dresses, a nude-colored shoe will also make your legs appear long.**

Shoes with a low vamp (the part of the shoe that covers the top of your foot); fitted knee-high boots; and pointy shoes will all elongate and slim the look of your ankles and legs. Chunky shoes and ankle straps make legs appear shorter.

If you have wide calves and have difficulty finding boots that fit, a good shoe repairman can insert a stretchy panel.

If you have heavy legs or thick ankles, stay away from ankle straps, flat shoes, ankle boots, and shoes with short delicate heels or high vamps.

Big women look better balanced in substantial shoes, but not too clunky. Wedge heels and the Sarah Palin special—open toes—are flattering.

Delicate women look better in delicate shoes.

---

too sexy

Height isn't everything. Comfort is supremely sexy. Toe cleavage is sexy. The narrower the heel, the sexier the shoe. Fabric, color, embellishments, and shape also make a sexy shoe.

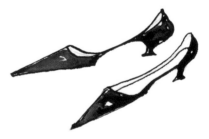

SEXY SHOES

If your body aches when you wear high heels, but not from desire, there are sexy alternatives. Fabric, color, pattern, embellishment, and cut contribute to shoe allure. Cutouts at the toe, sides, or back are sexy. Toe cleavage—shoes with a very low vamp to expose a bit of toes—is sexy. The narrower the heel is, the sexier the shoe. Knee-high narrow boots are sexy.

Closet Classics: Comfort Shoes

Belgian shoes. The Midinette is the original hand-sewn soft-soled classic Belgian loafer that was designed by Henri Bendel in the 1940s and remains the most popular. Those who wear them swear to their comfort and chic and collect them in a variety of patterns and color combinations.

Stubbs & Wootton handcrafted signature slipper shoes are renowed for their comfort and distinctively decorative and amusing designs.

Manolo Blahnik. The Carolyne two-inch slender-heeled pump remains a constant classic in his collections. They are the epitome of comfort, ageless style, and sexy elegance.

Cole Haan Nike Air pumps (and boots) and **Taryn Rose** (a Beverly Hills–based company founded by an orthopedic surgeon) were each worn by Angelina Jolie at the Cannes Film Festival when she was very pregnant with twins.

Ferragamo. The Vara, a solid low-heel pump with a grosgrain bow, has been Ferragamo's best-selling shoe since 1978. It remains a Closet Classic for women who want a low stylish heel for comfort and propriety.

Birkenstocks have an indentation in the heel, which reduces pressure on the ball of the foot. A ridge at the toes makes it easy for toes to grip when walking, and a roomy toe area allows feet to spread into their natural relaxed position.

Clogs. Those who spend much time on their feet (chefs, nurses) favor clogs because they are designed to reduce the stress on feet and backs. They are available in fashionable colors and patterns. Those by Dansko and Merrell are Closet Classics.

Pumas are sneakers that are sleeker looking than athletic shoes, and come in fashionable colors and textures, which makes them a favorite casual shoe outside the gym.

Uggs are those cozy suede boots from Australia that feel like slippers and keep your feet warm when you need it. There are many less expensive adaptations now available.

Closet Confidential: Reboot

"I wear cowboy boots because they are incredibly beautiful, handmade, I can find a variety that fit my size 11 feet, and I like what they say: *She's her own person.* I consider them my body armor. And they're also practical. I comfortably walked ten miles a day wearing them when I was on vacation in Rome, and I could hide my wallet in them."

Lise, fifty-four, attorney, Providence, Rhode Island

Dress for Your Height

My great-grandmother strapped a fork around my grandmother's waist so that if she slumped, she would be reminded to hold herself upright. Consequently my mother, sisters, and I were brought up with this family value when it would have been comforting to slouch to diminish our height (my youngest sister is six feet tall), especially during adolescence.

The better your posture, the trimmer and younger you will look, and the better your clothes will hang on your body.

After years of dressing, you likely know by now the dos and don'ts of dressing for your height. I am just shy of five foot ten and know that I don't need the lift of high heels, that wide-open necklines balance my long legs, and that short jackets are out of the question.

Shorter women likely know by now that short fitted jackets are more flattering than those that are longer and boxy. Knee-length skirts, narrow pants without pleats, vertical necklines, and monochromatic colors give the illusion of height. Belted jackets shorten your torso, as do cropped pants. Voluminous clothes, big accessories, and large details like wide lapels, big pockets, and oversize prints overwhelm your physique. It's better to reveal a part of your body so you don't look lost in your clothes— even three-quarter-length sleeves make a big difference.

As we get older, we shrink an average of two to three inches. Once osteoporosis sets in, our spinal column compresses, which means we all need to rethink the sizing, fit, and proportions of what we wear. This is likely why so many of us complain that it's difficult to find clothes that fit. We haven't adjusted to our changing body.

For many, **petite clothing** is a solution. There are many misconceptions about who should be wearing such sizing. We generally think one has to be five foot two or shorter. But petite sizing is not all about height.

Marcia, five foot six, was flabbergasted to learn from a personal shopper that her short arms and short waist made her a perfect candidate to shop for tops and jackets in the petite department. There she discovered jackets and sleeves that were cropped to suit her body. She was fifty-one and had never realized that regular-size jackets fell too low on her hips, causing the excess fabric to bunch around her midriff and add unnecessary bulk.

Didi is four inches shorter than Marcia, but long-waisted, so regular-size tops are better for her.

Andy, five six, is long-legged and short-waisted, with hips not much wider than her waist. She suspects that French women are petite because pants by French designers fit her body best. Otherwise she buys them in the boys' and men's department and has the waist taken in.

Despite your height or weight, if sleeves, hemlines, or waists run long, or if coats and jackets overwhelm your body, petite tops or bottoms might be a solution. It's all about body proportions.

Many are frustrated that petite styles are often dowdy or cutesy, rather than hip or stylish. Which is why some shop for simple classics and fresh looks in the children's department or stylish European children's stores. The fit is often a bit sexier, too.

Jeans are a challenge for petite-size women, but several women have recommended Levi's 515 Nouveau. Designer jeans are often cut long, so it's necessary to have them hemmed, then resewn to look like the original. It's pricey, but may work within your budget if you're buying other clothes in the kids department.

Dress for Your Curves, Whatever Their Shape

Look for Style Mentors with similar body types—Queen Latifah, Marilyn Monroe, Martha Stewart, Oprah—and study what they wear.

The worst thing you can do if you're extra-curvy is to wear boxy clothes. They'll just hang on your body, making it appear bigger and boxier.

Body shapers mask unwanted lumps.

High necklines are unflattering. Play up your shoulders with portrait and V-necklines.

Stay away from large prints and clothes that have a puffy silhouette.

Sheath and wrap dresses will play up your curves. A princess-cut dress or coat is also flattering.

Fabrics should caress, not cling, or be gutsy enough to hold shape.

A tailored tunic over boot-cut pants will create a balance that is flattering.

If you have an hourglass figure, the best thing you can do is to play it up! Dresses and skirts cut with curved seams embellish a svelte, hourglass figure.

Pencil skirts should taper at the knee and caress your bum.

Full skirts show off your waist—but stay away from puffy skirts.

Fitted strapless dresses are sexy. Be sure excess flesh doesn't protrude over the top.

Halter tops accentuate an hourglass figure.

Show off your waist with a jacket that is belted or cinched.

15

If You're Dressing Your Age, How Young Are You?

When there is an incompatibility between the style and a certain state of mind, it is never the style that triumphs.
—Coco Chanel

A few years before the Alien became full-blown, the man I had been dating asked me to dress sexy for our Valentine's Day lunch. What a fun thought. I pulled out my shortest skirt, which should have been recycled years before to my daughters' closet. I topped it with a Chinese-inspired blouse that said *exotic*—as did what I like to call my "tango shoes," worn with the requisite thigh-high fishnets. I ventured out on that rainy afternoon covered in another way-too-short but fabulous black silky trench coat with a leopard-print lining. From the moment I left the privacy of my home, I felt like *sex*, and it didn't feel sexy. Worse, I felt piercing eyes judging me as a "cash pickup" at the rather elegant, yet stuffy Upper East Side, New York, hotel restaurant where we dined.

Some would argue this is the stuff of fantasies, especially on the one day Cupid is obliged to release arrows of love, desire, or at least a fun flirt. *What pressure!* For me, though, what I wore crushed any notion of those feelings. I felt playful getting dressed earlier, but when I went public I felt like an imposter. I had confused sex with sexy. And let's face it: If you don't feel sexy, forget sex. My date thought I looked wow, but my mood dogged it all.

Unfortunately the clothes I wore to that Valentine's lunch should have been dejunked long ago. Clothes talk, and mine were saying *Get back into your closet and start recycling*. **The stuff of dreams became just stuff.**

Closet Confidential: License to Wear

"I have my clothes for a long time. I liked wearing my tight jeans with big square-toed boots and a leather jacket. It was my style, but lately it feels off. I asked my grown daughter what she thought and she confirmed that it looked terrible. We have an expression for this in Spanish: *Algunas veces mi ropa me desconoce*, which means 'My clothes don't recognize me.' I now feel estranged from some of my own clothes!"

Doris, forty-nine, construction company owner, Queens, New York

---

Finding Age-Appropriate Clothes in Your Closet

There is no single defining moment when certain things in our closet no longer feel age-appropriate to wear. There are lots of moments when we start to wonder *if*, or notice *yikes!* We all want to look great, but that doesn't mean like we did twenty years ago, or even ten years ago. Nor should we look like we've given up. Dowdy is dumb.

A few winters ago, I took my daughters to St. Barth's for a holiday. The seductive French island boasts celebrities and pristine beaches where, in the true French spirit of *laissez-faire*, the old, the young, the fat, and the fit relax side by side topless or in full monty. I was not comfortable baring all in front of my children, my sister's boyfriend, and his pubescent children, so I did the next best thing and wore a two-piece. Anything more and I would have felt as though I were hiding in a snowsuit. This was a time when the Alien was budding, but regardless, I felt relaxed with the beach culture there, which was about being comfortable with your body, whatever stage it was in. When my daughters protested that I was wearing too little, I told them it was the two-piece or no piece, which quieted them down until I emerged from the water not realizing my swimsuit had become completely transparent. I should have known better. Unless well lined, white swimsuits are revealing when wet. It mysteriously vanished after we returned to the hotel.

That day on the beach made me feel proud of me and all the other folks my age and older that we weren't hiding our changing bodies. But a beach on St. Barth's is one thing, the reality of everyday life is another. As we redefine our self-image, the question that haunts our closets is *What does age-appropriate mean for me now?* It's tricky, because there are no well-defined rules, and everyone else seems to have an opinion as to how we should look.

The cultural benchmarks that defined our mothers' generation don't apply as we continue to redefine what "age" looks and feels like. They grew up with rigid dress codes that marked each stage of their lives. We broke the rules. They wore girdles and stockings when we burned our bras—even if now we're wearing them again, not to mention the body-sculpting underpinnings that fill our closets. Jeans were to our mothers the clothes that cowboys and blue-collar laborers worked in. For us they were the legs of revolution, until they became a ubiquitous signature of everyday style—our new little black dress, although we've kept that, too.

We feel young and strong. We exercise, are responsible for putting *locavore* in the dictionary, and have chosen to be more independent than our mothers. They wore color-coordinated "outfits," while we learned to express our individuality by mixing things up.

Despite the fact that we redefined the rules of what was considered appropriate dressing decades ago, our children aren't shy about weighing in with their opinions of how we should and should not look now. My daughters were horrified when their forty-five-year-old aunt had her belly button pierced. They have vowed to remove theirs when they become mothers. They think it's inappropriate when women over forty wear sexy shirts with stylish jeans tucked into boots. Of course they couldn't wear jeans wherever they want today if it weren't for our generation. And they hate when mothers borrow their daughters' clothes. My daughter Carolyn and her friends tell me, "We want our mothers to be role models, rather than trying to look like our generation." Nevertheless, my girls still want me to look good. As Glenna shared, "Guys check out moms to see how their daughters might age."

MILF is a term used by young men for older mothers they desire (Mothers I'd Like to F**k).

Our children are critical when we err by dressing too young, but they also keep us from becoming dowdy.

Closet Confidential: *Growing Pretty*

"My mom and I have an ongoing war about how she dresses. She wears more conservative looks than she needs to. She's not comfortable dressing in a sexy or even feminine manner, because she never got the encouragement to show her sexuality and now lacks the confidence. She doesn't realize that it's okay to look pretty, sensual, and strong. Her clothes are a form of safety. I encourage her to try new things like skirts to the knee instead of mid-calf to show off her figure a bit—she has nice legs! I think because of my influence, she's now trying to look pretty. Clothes can look good on any body type if you believe in yourself and have the right attitude."

Karen, forty-three, retail consultant, Berkeley, California

What Does Age-Appropriate Mean to Us Now?

AGE-APPROPRIATE IS FINDING A BALANCE. We don't want to dress like our mothers *or* our daughters. Either extreme looks old to others and feels old to us. Hilary, a stylish forty-five-year-old magazine executive, sums it up: "It's unattractive to compete with twenty-year-olds, but I won't dress in a dull or matronly way. I dress to accentuate my positives. I'll wear skirts to show off my legs, but an inch above the knee, not a mini like I might have years ago."

AGE-APPROPRIATE IS TRUSTING YOUR GUT, NOT YOUR FEARS. To Susan, a West Marin mother of four young children, "I recently did a major purge of all the dowdy-looking clothes I owned, most of which my mother had given me. I had kept them for years thinking I would wear them when I turned fifty. Fifty came and went, and I realized they still looked dowdy and I didn't."

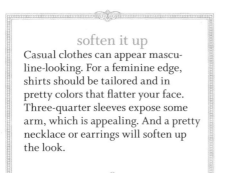

soften it up
Casual clothes can appear masculine-looking. For a feminine edge, shirts should be tailored and in pretty colors that flatter your face. Three-quarter sleeves expose some arm, which is appealing. And a pretty necklace or earrings will soften up the look.

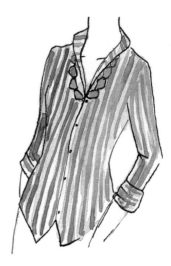

AGE-APPROPRIATE IS BEING MINDFUL OF YOUR BODY CHANGES AND RETHINKING WHAT YOU WEAR TO FLATTER THEM. To Andrea, a fifty-plus business executive, this means "not showing my arms, not bulging out of dresses, not showing the cleavage I used to have, wearing a sarong with my bathing suit, and changing my makeup to add more color to my skin."

AGE-APPROPRIATE IS BEING AWARE OF WHAT YOUR CLOTHES ARE SAYING.

My ex-boyfriend likes when women wear man-tailored shirts in fun colors, but I realized that with my high-energy and height (six feet) I can come across as aggressive and manly in them. I need a softer look, like tops with a scoop neck.
—Jill, fifty, Long Island, New York

AGE-APPROPRIATE IS DRESSING TO FEEL COMFORTABLE WITH YOURSELF. There was an interview in the August 2003 issue of American *Vogue* with Sarah Jessica Parker after she became a mother, which captured how naturally what we wear changes as we do: "I would never dress the way I dressed two years ago. I wouldn't even feel comfortable dressing the way I dressed a year ago, because I don't physically feel like I'm in the kind of shape that warrants wearing a particular dress or skirt . . . And it's not just a question of being in shape. A mother shouldn't run around town in low-slung jeans. I know we live in America and the Taliban aren't running this country . . . For me it's not right. It hasn't suited me for quite a while. I still want to feel like somebody would think I looked sexy or attractive. But I think it's a confirmation for women when they've had a baby: how they feel, how they want to feel."

AGE-APPROPRIATE IS WEARING JEANS AT ANY AGE, BUT NOT NECESSAR-ILY YOUR DAUGHTER'S JEANS. Theirs can trend to extremes—low-cut, exaggerated leg, skinny leg, embellished, distressed—while we need to focus on a flattering fit, denim with a bit of stretch and, unless we're wear-ing them to garden or clean the house, in darker colors—black, true blue, dark blue—and in white, all of which are Closet Classics.

> *I wonder what is age-appropriate, especially when I'm seated wearing low-slung jeans. I also wouldn't wear the lingerie look without a jacket anymore.*
> —Kathy, forty-five, interior decorator, San Francisco

Wear jeans with stylish shoes or boots for a polished, up-to-date look. Save the sneakers for workout clothes unless they're designed for style rather than exercise, like Pumas.

The fit of jeans should not be baggy or too tight, especially around the bum. If you are in between sizes, err on the smaller side, because jeans tend to give with wear. A better option, however, is to try on other styles. You must be able to sit comfortably; the waistline should not be very low (too young) or belted at the waist (dowdy), but fall somewhere just below your belly button depending on your build. Try on several different styles. You'll know when you get it right.

Boot-cut legs are Closet Classics, because they are the most versatile to pair with a variety of clothes and shoes, and are the most flattering for most body types. The slight flare of the leg balances a thick middle and wide hips.

The smaller the rear pockets, the larger your bum will appear.

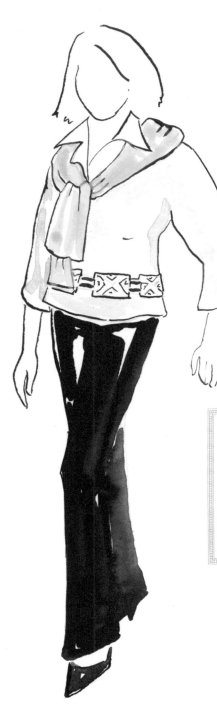

> ### Caring Closet
>
> If your jeans need to be hemmed, wash them first. To keep denim dark, and maintain denim that has stretch, wash jeans in cold water and dry on a low cycle.

AGE-APPROPRIATE IS NOT BARING YOUR MIDRIFF, no matter how toned you are, unless you are exercising, on a beach, in bed, or having sex.

Age-appropriate is covering your tattoos and belly ring, and not baring lots of cleavage or your midriff. Strapless tops are only appropriate if your arms are in good shape. Leggings should only be worn by the young and thin. Crocs only look good on children. Tie-less Converse sneakers should only be worn at home. And shorts should not be worn in the city.
—Terry, forty-six, financial consultant, Manhattan

AGE-APPROPRIATE IS DRESSING FOR PHYSICAL COMFORT, BUT NOT GIVING UP ON STYLE. As Teresa, a social worker in New York City, says, "I love comfort, but not ugly." There is nothing attractive about teetering in stilettos if it's difficult to walk, or fabrics that don't feel good against the skin in the throes of a hot flash. There are other stylish options available—decorative flats, fabrics designed to wick away moisture, or dressing in layers.

AGE-APPROPRIATE IS KNOWING THAT NO MATTER HOW BUFF YOU ARE, TIGHT IS TOO TIGHT. Clothes that fit and caress your curves will show off your body at its best.

AGE-APPROPRIATE IS KNOWING THAT DRESSING TO FLATTER YOUR BODY TAKES PRECEDENCE OVER WEARING A TREND. Always. No matter how beautiful something appears on a hanger, in a picture, or on someone else, if it looks like it's wearing you, feels uncomfortable, or doesn't play up your assets, it's not for you.

AGE-APPROPRIATE IS MASKING VISIBLE NIPPLE ERECTION. If you hate wearing a bra, wear pasties.

AGE-APPROPRIATE IS KNOWING THAT IT IS ENTIRELY YOUR DECISION WHETHER OR NOT TO BARE YOUR ARMS. Jill Biden, Caroline Kennedy, Diane von Furstenberg, Goldie Hawn, and Glenn Close continue to bare theirs. It's Michelle Obama's style signature even in the chill of winter.

Some hate the sight of their underarm jiggles; others couldn't care less. Our mothers' generation seemed less concerned with this issue than does ours. Many women who have toned arms want to show them off. Others prefer to cover them up whatever their age. Either way, it's about your comfort zone.

> ## Closet Confidential: Disarming
>
> "Age-appropriate has some meaning for me. For example, I wear sleeveless, but my husband and I went to a birthday dinner recently and the hostess (fifty) wore a sleeveless dress but had underarm jiggles, which were accentuated every time she toasted. It was distracting!"
>
> *Susan, fifty-two, design entrepreneur, Manhattan*

AGE-APPROPRIATE IS TURNING YOUR FAVORITE MINI SKIRTS INTO PILLOWS, REGARDLESS OF HOW GREAT YOUR LEGS ARE. Even supermodel Cindy Crawford expressed her reservations in British *Vogue*: "I'm 38 and if I wear a mini, it's only on the beach." If you insist, wear them with dark opaque tights. It will soften the issue of hemline. The most appropriate and flattering length for skirts is mid-knee. If your legs are an asset, accentuate them with great shoes, boots, or patterned hosiery.

AGE-APPROPRIATE IS BEING MINDFUL OF HOW YOU BARE YOUR LEGS. If you choose to go bare-legged, play down veins, broken capillaries, and uneven pigmentation with a self-tanner, leg makeup, or even nude-colored fishnet hosiery—which are age-appropriate when balanced by an otherwise classic look.

I dress for fun; however, I know that even though I am a size zero, I cannot dress like I am twenty! I do not wear shorts at all, but I do wear Capris and cropped pants. I believe you simply must leave a little for the imagination!
—Brenda, fifty, executive assistant, Frisco, Texas

AGE-APPROPRIATE IS REPLACING YOUR LEATHER PANTS WITH SUEDE, unless you're going for the bondage look. Otherwise leather is appropriate when worked in classic shapes—trench, simple skirt, vest, blazer—and worn with contrasting fabrics, say a cashmere sweater.

AGE-APPROPRIATE IS NOT LOOKING DOWDY. Try on new ideas. Add a surprise element to what you are wearing—a jazzy shoe, a jacket with an edgy cut, fun earrings.

AGE-APPROPRIATE IS KNOWING THAT IF YOU WORE A TREND THE FIRST TIME IT CAME AROUND, NOT TO WEAR IT AGAIN. Many of us first started wearing fashion in the 1960s and '70s when mini skirts, baby-doll dresses, and peasant shirts were the rage. But now decades later, are they still appropriate for us to wear even when stores are packed with clothes influenced by these retro styles? Nothing will make us look older than wearing trends from our youth that are marketed to our daughters. If you are passionate about wearing a vintage piece you already own, mix it with Closet Classics for balance.

Closet Confidential: *Timely or Timeless*

"Because I started out as a fashion copywriter at *Harper's Bazaar* in the very hip, very cool 1960s, I still pay attention to what's in and what's out. I was literally trained by the more senior editors and photographers I worked with not only to live in the now but to pay attention to the nextness of things—to be curious and perpetually tuned in to changes and nuances of style; to pay attention to whatever was the upcoming, fresh, or even revolutionary in affecting all aspects of our culture.

"I never slavishly followed fashion, but by trying on different types of clothes, I did learn more about my own body—what works and what doesn't. So now I know there are some things I shall never revisit. No more grommets or tough-looking hardware-type zippers; suede yes, black leather no; never again mini skirts; and those chic lady-like bow-tied silk blouses that looked so professional under suits when I was in my early forties, and are having another run in fashion today, would look positively dowdy on me the second time around. These days I prefer the streamlined versus anything too embellished, too ruffled, complicatedly cut, overly ethnic in inspiration, or too obviously body revealing."

Kathryn, sixty-five, writer, Manhattan

AGE-APPROPRIATE IS GOING FOR QUALITY OVER TREND.

I wear the best I can afford, and if I can't afford it, I buy it anyway and make it last longer—I don't care about changing looks. Good clothes are made better. They have better lines and design, and really do fit better.

—Betsy, sixty-four, Ketchum, Idaho

Clothes made in the 1920s or before are considered antique. Those made between the 1920s and 1980s are considered vintage, and those between 1965 and 1985 are often referred to as retro. More recent designs are contemporary or modern.

AGE-APPROPRIATE IS KNOWING WHEN OUR BODIES ARE CHANGING, NOT TO HIDE IN BOXY OR SHAPELESS CLOTHES. They look old and careless on us now.

The biggest mistake after I gained weight in menopause was wearing baggy clothes. They just made me look bigger.

—Marilyn, sixty-plus, Internet entrepreneur, Chatham, New York

Even Eileen Fisher and Chico's, two fashion houses known for designing comfortable and stylish clothes for "real" bodies, have added shape to their collection with subtle seams and a bit of stretch, and by playing with proportion.

If you wear something roomy, counter it with something more fitted or tailored, and always add an attractive element to spruce up the look— jazzy shoes, fun earrings, a colorful scarf. It combines style and comfort and shows you haven't given up on yourself.

AGE-APPROPRIATE IN HOT WEATHER IS WEARING A SUNDRESS WITH THE OPTION OF COVERING YOUR ARMS with a lightweight wrap, cardigan, or jacket with three-quarter-length sleeves in a light color so it looks summery.

Closet Confidential: *Those Were the Days*

"I have moments of mourning what I looked like when I see pictures of the young me, especially in a bikini. I was always complaining about the way I looked, but realize now I would love to look that way. I now have cellulite on my thighs so will only wear a bathing suit with a sarong. I don't like my arms now, but I've accepted them and wear three-quarter-length sleeves even on the hottest summer days."

Andrea, fifty-plus, business executive, Manhattan

AGE-APPROPRIATE IS WEARING A ONE-PIECE SWIMSUIT (black!) that performs like a body shaper. An attractive beach cover-up makes the ordeal look chic.

AGE-APPROPRIATE IS NO LONGER WEARING SHORT-SHORTS unless you're working out. Age-appropriate alternatives are tailored shorts cut to the knee or Capri pants.

White pants are summer Closet Classics. Be sure panties and body lumps are not visible. With unlined pants, wear nude panties that match your skin color. Thigh-length body shapers will smooth out cellulite. Remove pocket liners if visible.

AGE-APPROPRIATE IS NOT WEARING HEAD-TO-TOE MATCHING DESIGNER CLOTHES, or matching earrings with a necklace or bracelet, or shoes with a bag. It looks dowdy. When this 1950s fashion moment is revived, as all trends are, leave it to your children to play with. They can get away with it; we can't.

AGE-APPROPRIATE IS NOT WEARING SOUVENIR T-SHIRTS except for gardening or sleeping in, unless they're vintage rock and roll and fitted. Otherwise you look unkempt.

AGE-APPROPRIATE IS KNOWING THAT IF YOU QUESTION WHETHER WHAT YOU ARE WEARING IS AGE-APPROPRIATE, CHANCES ARE IT'S NOT.

None of us want to look ridiculous, which means not looking like the latest trend, or wearing lots of busy patterns. Young girls are able to get away with that, but simpler lines and patterns are better for adults.
—Diane, sixty-four, design writer, Manhattan

AGE-APPROPRIATE IS DRESSING FOR YOUR OWN PLEASURE. It's knowing the rules, and knowing you can break them.

CONFIDENCE IS THE BEST THING YOU CAN WEAR AT ANY AGE.

16

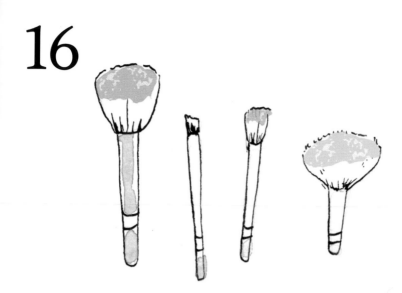

Are You Wearing Your Best Face?

Beauty is only skin-deep, but so are wrinkles, sun spots, broken capillaries—need I go on? Denial or not, most of us have a clue that our face, neck, and hair are in transition, but **even the queen in** Snow White and the Seven Dwarfs **had to ask her mirror each morning for a reality check.** I had gotten so distracted by the Alien that I hadn't noticed changes in my face until my daughters expressed their terror that I might have skin cancer. The healthy glow I saw in the mirror was a scary inferno to others.

Upon closer examination, I realized that my eyebrows were becoming dangerously sparse, and I was never a plucker! I had already accepted that my eyelashes would no longer curl, even with the gold standard of eyelash curlers by Shu Uemura, but now they were also disappearing at the outer edges of my eyes. Ugh! What next? Was I also applying makeup like "those" older women who wear beauty masks in their attempts to remain frozen in time? Norma Desmond is not my idea of beauty.

> In the 1950 Billy Wilder movie Sunset Boulevard, Norma Desmond was a delusional faded movie star played by Gloria Swanson, shielded from the reality that she was no longer the young beauty she once was. Wishful thinking. Be careful to stay away from lip liners and heavy facial makeup. Apply as little as possible to specific targets, and absolutely say no to brilliantly colored or frosted eye shadows. And choose which zone to play up—eyes or lips. Otherwise you may not be shielded, like Norma, from looking older than you need to.

Now that my attention was diverted from the Alien, I started to catch glimpses of my fuller face and weaker jawline—another legacy of my dad I thought I had taken care of with a little lipo under the chin in my forties when my professional appearance seemed important. **I thought I was too young for jowls!** They clashed with my self-identity. But that procedure, like all cosmetic surgery, has an expiration date, and my time was clearly up. My body to-do list was growing faster than a woman's unwanted facial hair. I needed an overhaul, but where to start?

> Pay attention to your grooming: hair, makeup, nails. Do your teeth need
> whitening? How about facial hair? As a friend's father commented: "The
> older I get, the less whiskers I have, and the more they appear on my lady
> friends' faces." They may be subtle, so do a mirror check in bright light from
> all angles.

To appease my daughters, I checked in with my dermatologist, Dr.
Linda Franks. My stars had aligned: The piling on of recent stress, a lifetime of sun abuse, rapidly changing hormones, and my Nordic heritage
all contributed to my diagnosis: rosacea.

> Rosacea is a skin condition characterized by reddening, dilated blood vessels,
> stinging skin, or bumps that sometimes resemble pimples. It is more common in
> women of Celtic or Northern European descent between the ages of thirty
> and fifty. Outbreaks can be triggered by alcohol, caffeine, stress, wind,
> dramatic changes in temperature, vigorous exercise, spicy foods, and sun.
> Sometimes rosacea is mistaken for acne. Acne products will aggravate the
> condition. See your dermatologist and stick to over-the-counter products
> designed to cleanse and moisturize sensitive skin. My favorite find is organic
> sesame oil, an antioxidant that penetrates the skin deeper than any other oil. I
> use it regularly to nourish my face and my body (www.youthingstrategies.com).

I had just read in *The New York Times* that facial redness was the new
cellulite. Lovely. There is no escaping it. I am so typical of my generation,
one in which we all felt so unique! Despite advances in cosmetic surgery
and skin rejuvenation, there is no cure for rosacea. It was now part of the
landscape of my face for the rest of my life. Dr. Linda Franks gave me a
quick education on what type of skin products to use and to avoid, the
importance of wearing sunblock, a list of food and drinks to stay clear of,
and a couple of prescriptions and skin treatments to up the antioxidants
and halt (I hope) the condition from progressing further. While she was
at it, she also had my thyroid checked to see whether it was responsible for
my disappearing brows. Results: negative.

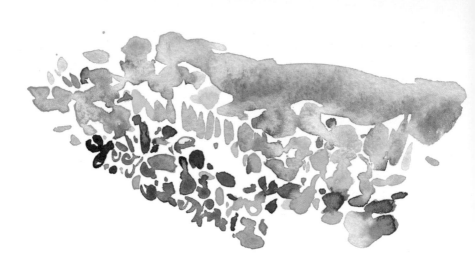

There are flowers everywhere for those who bother to look.
—Henri Matisse

I also needed to rethink my makeup. As our hormones scramble, our face betrays our genetics, stress, sun damage, and other naughty habits. Its coloring, texture, and contour change, and so must our skin regimen, the kinds of makeup we apply, and the way we apply it. If we're stuck in a beauty freeze, using the same skin care products or cosmetics we've been wearing for years, then we are simply not looking our best.

I made appointments at various cosmetic counters whose "brand look" was the natural I was hoping to achieve with my new condition. Most beauty counters in department stores offer free consultations along with an application of makeup by an expert. You may leave a session feeling overly made up, but it's likely that you've picked up a new technique or information so you can choose better when shopping for mass-market brands. The cosmetics industry is constantly developing better products specifically designed for our changing skin.

At one counter, I found a butter-yellow-based concealer that blended effortlessly over my red spots (yellow offsets redness) and under eye shadows. There were days when that was all I needed. For times when the flush was particularly brilliant, I found something a bit heavier that was a cross between concealer and foundation—again, very creamy to avoid a dry, caked look, and which I only applied to the areas of my face in need.

Now that I had to diligently protect my skin from the sun, a makeup artist at another counter gave me a *healthy*-looking sun-kissed glow by lightly dabbing a huge soft makeup brush into a bronzy-colored fine powder, then brushing it gingerly on my cheekbones, on my forehead, and a bit under my chin for the definition I longed for.

Another professional turned me on to a brow pencil that doesn't require sharpening (sharpeners always eat the end of my makeup pencils). **Brows give the face definition.** She *gently* feathered a slightly darker color of my hair onto my brow line. She also pointed out how the black eyeliner I had been using looked severe and that midnight blue was a softer alternative that would bring out the blue in my blue-green eyes.

Caring Closet
A magnifying mirror with attached lighting takes the guesswork out of applying makeup and checking for unwanted facial hair.

The big buzz at the counters was that **lashes are the new lips.** Translation: Cosmetically swollen lips were out, and long, lustrous lashes were in. And I wanted in! I spent a small fortune having an expert apply individual lashes, which achieved the desired lustrous effect, but lasted only a few weeks before shedding. There was no way I was going to add this luxury to my "maintenance" budget for the rest of my life. Another makeup artist turned me on to an eyelash conditioner (Cils Booster XL by Lancôme), which positively extended and curled my wispy, dull lashes. When I added mascara, they looked luxurious.

One of the gals behind a counter also turned me onto RevitaLash, a pricey product (cheaper online) that was developed by a doctor for his wife when she lost her lashes during chemotherapy. Allegedly, if used every day for three to four weeks, it accelerates the growth of lashes. I was astonished—it worked far better than I could have imagined! I was not alone. After several weeks of application, Diane, a sixty-four-year-old self-confessed magazine junkie up on the latest in everything, reported: "My daughter thought I was wearing false eyelashes!"

As I was getting the basics of my new face taken care of, I knew I also needed to take a fresh look at what I was wearing around my face.

Anything red now made my rosaceous face look even more red. Turtlenecks lit my inner furnace and emphasized my fuller face. And I wanted to add some pizzazz to my look, rather than dwell on the unwanted changes that were going on from the neck up. It was time for some Mirror Talk to figure out how to dress my new face.

Hot flashes and makeup. Beauty expert Liz Michael advised me that when you're experiencing a hot flash, go into a cooler room and lightly blot your face with tissue until it calms down. Do not powder your face, as it will clog with sweat and look uneven. Also, use the sheerest foundation for the most minimal coverage possible. The more transparent, the less havoc it will cause on the look of your makeup after a hot flash. Heavy products will look blotchy in the aftermath.

Old and new makeup. Don't pile on makeup to cover telltale signs of aging. The more foundation and powders you apply, the older your skin will look. Instead, change the kind of products you use. Stay away from matte or iridescent textures, which will emphasize wrinkles. Use those that are light and luminous. Dab on foundation or concealer only where you need it. If your skin texture has dulled, add some color with a tinted moisturizer or creamy blush. Eyebrows tend to fade over time, so softly darken them with a brow pencil or shadow in a color slightly darker than your original hair color. It will help to define your eyes and frame your face. Avoid bright lip colors, and choose those with moisturizer or gloss.

Dress Your Face

Pay attention to the colors you are wearing close to your face. As your skin tone changes, you will need to bring more light to your face with color and jewelry.

If you've become jowly, wrinkly, or droopy, wear something decorative near your face—distinctive glasses, dazzling earrings, an embellished neckline, or an eye-catching scarf. It will add interest away from what you perceive as new flaws.

Turtlenecks are tricky. For some, they are the perfect camouflage. For others, they make jowls look like they've been squeezed up and out through a tube of toothpaste. If going the turtleneck route, many of us do better with a cowl neck or unfitted turtleneck.

If you have a clean jawline (rejoice!), short hair, bangs, and long earrings will show it off.

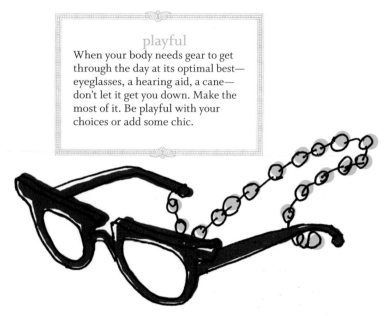

Glasses

Sometime after turning forty, almost every one of us will require reading glasses. If you're like me, you'll need a pair in your car, at your desk, and in every room of your home. There are times I wander around unknowingly wearing three pairs pushed back to the top of my head.

Rather than feeling the gloom of impending age, consider glasses an opportunity to accessorize your face. I spent a mini fortune on my first pair, which I bought at an eyeglass boutique. They were like a piece of sculpture—deep red and shaped like a pagoda. Instead of feeling old when I wore them, I felt cool. I now buy my reading glasses at bargain prices in whimsical shapes and colors at pharmacies, supermarkets, bookstores, airport newsstands, and even car washes.

Eyeglass chains are convenient for finding your glasses quickly, and glasses can be as pretty as a necklace or as sleek as your active gear. Just be sure that if you are big-breasted, they don't cascade over your front.

If you need to wear eyeglasses 24/7, make them an extension of your personal style. Think how Sarah Palin's Kazuo Kawasaki frame model

704, in color gray, became the rage during the 2008 presidential campaign. My local bank teller looks infinitely more fabulous now wearing a pair. One glamorous fashion editor I had long admired was unable to have a face-lift because of heart problems, so she took to wearing huge black glasses. They became her trademark and diverted attention from her aging face. If you're not into drama, choose glasses that contrast in shape with your face—a long, narrow face looks better with a horizontal or oval frame. Angular frames flatter round faces.

Sunglasses have long been associated with glamour, mystery, style, and sports. They also keep us from squinting, which exacerbates deep wrinkles. Most importantly, sunglasses are critical for the good health of eyes that see the light of day, but only if they provide a wide span of UV protection. Anything less merely shades eyes, which dilates the pupils, allowing in harmful rays.

There are three types of UV rays, all of which are harmful and cause cataracts and other eye diseases. UVA penetrates the deepest, UVB inflicts the most damage, and UVC is the most powerful. There are also harmful blue light rays known as HEV (high-energy visible) that contribute to glare and can lead to macular degeneration. Large wraparound glasses (look at Jackie O and Audrey), shield eyes best from the sun and look as fabulous worn with high fashion as they do near high surf.

Southern beauties have long known the chic of wearing hats and their importance in protecting their renowned youthful-looking skin from harmful UV rays. Whether you wear them in cold weather for warmth or in hot weather for sun protection, to salvage a bad hair day or simply for the fun of it, hats provide a frame for dressing your face. Choices can be as casual as a baseball cap or as decorative as those worn by ladies attending the Royal Ascot. For serious sun protection, wear hats and clothes made from fabric that provides UV protection.

Wearing reading glasses is one thing, but a hearing aid? There is no way our age-phobic youthquake generation wants to figure this into the equation of redefining our self-image.

We grew up with rock and roll—loud rock and roll. About one in six boomers have hearing loss. There are more of us between the ages of forty-five and sixty-five with hearing loss (ten million) than those over sixty-five (nine million). So much for good vibrations. And I thought my daughters were merely mumbling and that my cell phone didn't get good reception—anywhere! And did you know that if all noise is blocked when you're listening to your iPod, or if others can hear what you're listening to, the volume is causing damage to your hearing?

Tuning out is old. Thankfully the hearing industry is one of the many industries anticipating our changing physical and self-image requirements. Today some hearing aids can be mistaken for an iPod or cell phone, and combine wireless and Bluetooth connectivity to streamline cell phone calls. There are models that look like a groovy earring in animal prints, psychedelic colors, or—for the luxe consumer—alligator. And if you can't imagine a hearing aid being the new head jewelry, there's a device that could become the contact lenses of hearing aids—invisible to the eye.

According to the Better Hearing Institute, research indicates that those with untreated hearing loss experience depression, anxiety, fatigue, and short-term memory loss. They also earn less money than their counterparts with hearing aids. So get with it, rather than be out of it.

A Word About Wrinkles

She looks like she got her looks from her father. He's a plastic surgeon. —Groucho Marx

Early in my career as a fashion editor at *Town & Country* magazine, I wrote copy and styled photo shoots, but wanted to learn how to put all the elements together on a page, which is what designers in magazine art departments do. After a few years, I left *T&C*, much to my mother's chagrin at the time, to study graphic design at Parsons School of Design.

I needed to find a part-time job to help support this pursuit. I got a job in the art department of Peter Rogers Associates, an advertising agency that specialized in award-winning fashion and beauty campaigns including, *What Becomes a Legend Most?*, which featured famous celebrities swathed in Blackglama minks.

When the "legends" dropped by the agency (Claudette Colbert, Liza Minnelli, Rudolf Nureyev, and Faye Dunaway to name a few), Peter Rogers, the charismatic owner, would introduce them to all of us who worked there. A legendary story told in the art department was how Lauren Bacall chastised the art department for retouching the wrinkles out of her portrait. She was proud of them. I was only twenty-five at the time, but it left a lifelong impression on me. I admired her wish to keep them as testament to a life rich in experiences rather than having them erased. Culturally we are trained to see wrinkles and think *old*, while Bacall claimed they were emblematic of living.

There are many cosmetic remedies that diminish wrinkles, from creams to silicone injections to cosmetic acupuncture. Botox has been popular for its ability to paralyze the muscles that exacerbate wrinkles, but the result can be in stark contrast with an aging neck or hands. Fountain-of-youth options will continue to grow as our culture remains youth-obsessed. It's all about priorities. Some women are appalled at being injected with poison, while for others it's as routine as a manicure. Some feel it's a necessary line item in their budget; others would rather spend the money to pay off their mortgage or save for retirement or an experience they can share with others. Some feel it's important for their appearance in the workplace or in their marriage. Others prefer a holistic approach to their beauty.

More Magazine reported:

> *Almost three-quarters of cosmetic surgery is done on patients under 50 years old. Seems a funny thing happens after we hit that big birthday: We relax. Surveys consistently show that post 50; we're happier, more confident and more socially involved than younger women.*

One gal told me that her forty-year-old friend had a nip and tuck with results that put her into hiding—even from her good friends—for close to a year until her face settled. "Can you imagine losing a year of your life that way?" she asked.

Glamorous Andrea who spends a small fortune on cosmetic procedures remains conflicted on having a face-lift. Some friends who went through the procedure had unattractive results.

Betsy, a fit sixty-four-year-old, defines *old* as women whose faces and bodies don't match in age.

Hilary, an attractive forty-five-year-old magazine executive, says: "I have a burning desire for an eye job, but I'm too chicken and too cheap for surgery. Besides my friends and husband know what I look like."

For me, I am not as concerned about wrinkles as I am about having my chin cleaned up, which falls somewhere on my burgeoning to-do list after paying off credit card debt and losing twenty pounds of menopausal weight. Meanwhile, I need to dress my face by also rethinking the colors I wear to frame it.

However we choose to regard our wrinkles or droopiness, we need to understand that cosmetic procedures will not create a spirit of youthfulness. There are eighty-year-olds with a girlish spark, just as there are thirty-year-olds without.

Wrinkles reflect your life and personality. I can't say that I'm proud of them, but they are there. It's an irreversible process, and once you accept that, then you feel better within yourself. —French model Françoise de Staël, seventy-four

Beauty Closet

I spend more money now on my skin—facials, moisturizers, eye cream—because once your skin goes, it's gone. I want to maintain what I have. —Jill, fifty, Long Island, New York

In a study in the *American Journal of Clinical Nutrition,* scientists scrutinized the skin of four thousand people and found that **those who consumed more vitamin C had significantly fewer wrinkles** than those with a lower intake. Lead study author Maeve Cosgrove, PhD, reported that the antioxidant properties may help boost the production and regeneration of collagen—the protein that keeps skin supple.

Sleep is the best beauty treatment you can give yourself. A few of the many benefits of a good night's sleep are that it reduces stress and inflammation, which is thought to contribute to our body's aging process. Stress can impair the skin's barrier function, which keeps bacteria out and water in. Studies show that the skin of people in chronic stress healed slower. Stress can contribute to flare-ups of alopecia areata (a form of hair loss), and skin diseases like psoriasis and eczema. Strive for at least six hours; eight hours is ideal.

17

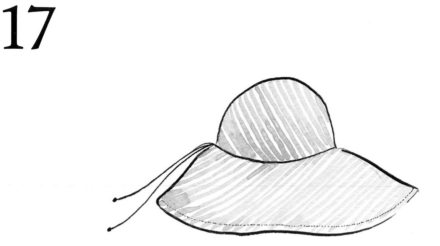

Locks in Time

For most of my life, I have worn my blond hair long and straight. Until I turned forty, I maintained the highlights with a mix of lemon juice and summer sun, later with chemicals. It's my look. Easy to manage and maintain.

When I was a young working woman, I marked the end of the summer trial live-in I had with my then husband-to-be by walking into a renowned hair salon off Fifth Avenue and asking the stylist to cut off all my hair. The results could only be described as Peter Pan–like—boyishly short. I then dressed for my new hair by wearing very feminine clothes so there would be no mistaking my sex or sexuality. As shocked as everyone who knew me was, I felt strangely liberated. It was as if I was challenging the depth or criteria upon which relationships are built. I had considered my hair a metaphor for youth's transient beauty and confidence. *Will you, will I, still love me even when my youthful appearance fades as my body unfolds in ways I can't know?*

In your twenties, people get married for passion, in your thirties, it's for children, in your forties, it's for money and prestige. But in your fifties, you want someone who would go through chemotherapy with you. So that's what I'd like—to find someone who would love me without my hair.
—Suzy Kellett, quoted in *Fifty on Fifty* by Bonnie Miller Rubin

I eventually married this man and grew my hair back into its signature look. But when the marriage fell apart, I once again relinquished my hair to a professional. "You're here for the divorce cut," he remarked. Apparently it's not uncommon for women to alter their hair when experiencing a dramatic life shift. It's the quickest and most dramatic change we can make when we're in the process of redefining ourselves and reimagining the rest of our lives. It's like shedding a skin—a fresh start. And it's the easiest to salvage if we don't like the results.

Closet Confidential: Lighten Up

"After my husband passed away, I had the choice of being a victim and bitter, or try to enjoy life again. I decided to look on the Internet for a new partner. I met with my first 'victim,' who suggested that it might be nicer for me to change my very classical (stuffy) hairdo. I had it cut short and layered and put in blond highlights. I looked so much younger. I was motivated to lose ten pounds and buy some new clothes—shorter skirts because my legs are okay, skinny trousers, vests, and exciting boots! For the first time in many years I found the courage to spend money on myself, even though I had the resources before. I feel good about myself now—I found the new me. Actually it's the 'me' I had forgotten about. I do not see this man anymore but I am grateful to him for suggesting the haircut."

Cary, fifty-five, Amsterdam, the Netherlands

Hair is powerful. It's the stuff of fairy tales and legends. In Greek mythology, Medusa was a beautiful priestess in Athena's temple. After Poseidon raped her, Athena transformed Medusa's hair into serpents. If a man were to look at her, he would turn to stone. In Jewish law, the Talmud teaches that a woman's hair exudes sensual energy, and covering it ensures a married woman's modesty. And like the biblical Samson, many of us feel that we'll lose power if we lose the hair of our youth. Yet being held captive by hair is more about losing our power, not embracing it.

Closet Confidential: Wigged Out

When Paullette lost her hair during chemo, she bought wigs—lots of wigs. Her co-workers never knew who was going to show up in the morning. She was flirtatious as a blonde and strictly business in the brunette bob. She felt gutsy as a redhead, and her joy was infectious when she wore a blue-and-silver Dallas Cowboys wig.

Paullette's experience with cancer opened her up to taking more risks and having more fun in all aspects of her life. "I lost a lot of personal fear after facing death. I wanted to be more expressive whether it meant wearing more color or speaking up in the male-dominated office environment I worked in. It's funny; once I did, I got a substantial promotion."

Paullette, forty-plus, oil industry executive, San Antonio, Texas

W2W Closet Journal: Time for a Change?

Do you have bad hair days?

Has the coloring and texture of your hair changed?

When was the last time you changed the way you cared for it?

When was the last time you experimented with the way you wear your hair?

Is it time to shake things up and refresh your look?

The first step is making a change is always the most difficult. It means letting go of the familiar and allowing for the unknown: new successes and possibly new failures.

It's the ultimate freedom when we muster the courage to take a chance and experiment with our hair, rather than remain locked in time. Consider it a mid-life adventure. Why not?

Closet Confidential: *New Hair Day*

"I am going through a personal 'makeover.' At forty-four, I am changing inside and out and want to reflect that in my style. I am ready for fun. I'm even thinking about dying my hair red."

Martie, Lafayette, Louisiana

"I change my hair every three months. I'll go from a big 'fro to straight hair so I can wear cute hats in rainy or cold weather. I think it's old when you have the same style for years and years and years."

Karen, thirty-nine, executive editor, South Orange, New Jersey

"When I turned fifty, I cut my hair off in a bob style and started letting it dry naturally. It's so curly now. I love it!"

Brenda, fifty, executive assistant, Frisco, Texas

"I change my hairstyle every seven weeks. When you're comfortable with your stylist, you don't have to explain or justify. I tell mine to do what she wants within good taste. And I love the way a fun white streak has grown in the front of my naturally dark hair."

Beatriz, forty-nine, CEO of HispanAmérica and power yoga teacher, Newfoundland, Pennsylvania

"Moving to Alabama was an important passage in my life because I was in a very new place geographically and culturally (I'm originally from Chicago). My husband was traveling a lot for business, and my daughter was busy with her own life. I started wondering what would happen to me when everyone disappears. Art has always been an important part of my life, so I decided at this major turning point to get my master's in art history, and become very involved with the local museum. I still had a cute 'yummy mummy' figure as my husband calls it, but I started graying and found that no one was paying attention to me. So I kept my dark eyebrows and went platinum blond. My daughter was so embarrassed every time I picked her up from school, because I didn't look preppy like the other mothers. My husband got used to it. And I got attention!"

Julia, fifty-plus, art consultant, Richfield, Idaho

> "I've learned to challenge the 'beauty' laws I had long trusted. My husband took a consulting job in Peru, a Spanish-speaking country, and I don't speak Spanish. After settling us into a new home, I then had to take care of me. First on the list was a desperately needed trim. I had been religious about my blunt cut, believing it flattered best my very fine, straight hair. The hairdresser interpreted my visual attempts at communicating what I wanted by layering my hair in a very subtle way, which gave it infinitely more bounce, making it look more alive—I daresay, more youthful. I was lucky to have been forced to relinquish my control. Self-imposed style rules are good ideas for gross blunders, but not otherwise. It's good to shake yourself up!"
>
> *Marilyn, sixty-plus, Internet entrepreneur, Chatham, New York*

For my divorce cut, the stylist gave me bangs, which didn't flatter my round face and weak chin, but he also layered into my signature blunt cut, which was starting to become dull and flat looking. And for the first time I began using product—hair-thickening shampoo plus conditioner and spray for volume, which along with a quick upside-down blow dry and a few Velcro rollers livened up my layers with very little effort.

Hair Mentors

Just as we can learn from our Style Mentors, Hair Mentors can inspire us, too. I like short modern cuts with attitude like Annie Lennox's bleached white hair and Jamie Lee Curtis's natural gray. I am enamored with silver-white hair and the confidence of the women who wear it. I also love voluminous manes of natural curls that beautifully frame a face, and I think dreadlocks are way cool. I admire how some women have found an iconic look, like legendary *Vogue* editor Anna Wintour's perfect bob, which over the years has become lighter and subtly layered.

But over the years I also have gotten to know more about me and my hair. Short hair doesn't flatter my face or height—just shy of five ten. My hair is very straight, so curls are out. The last time I tried a permanent, I looked like a wet poodle. Besides my hair gurus—Jen Cloke and Edita Evon at the Warren-Tricomi Salon in Greenwich, Connecticut, tell me it is the worst thing you can do to your hair. I am not savvy at wielding a blow dryer with finesse, nor is it on my list of new things to accomplish in life. I have no interest in spending more time getting myself pulled together and out the door than I do now. I know that blond highlights bring out the best in my complexion, but I have them done subtly so I don't have to retouch them frequently. So for now, I am happy with my easy-to-care-for blond, layered, shoulder-length hair.

Jenny Cloke has been my colorist for more years than I can remember. It was hit or miss, mostly miss, until I luckily found her through my stylist Edita Evon. I found Edita through my friend Becky, whose trademark short turned-under cut suddenly had more movement thanks to Edita's magic. I went to her for some hair oomph, too! Both Jenny and Edita are with the Warren-Tricomi Salon in Greenwich, Connecticut.

Closet Confidential: Color Me, Me!

"I try on wigs in different colors, but continue to dye my hair organically with henna to keep it black. Everyone including my hairstylist tells me it looks too dark and to cut it shorter [it falls below her chest]. But I talk to myself and say, 'My long dark hair is my landmark.' It's the only thing I can't change my thinking about. I want to grow it even longer to my waist and wear it straight. I feel it makes me look young."

Doris, forty-nine, construction company owner, Queens, New York

I still look for Hair Mentors, but those whose hair is similar in color and texture to mine. For me it's Martha Stewart (suburban chic), Candace Bergen (modern, yet elegant grown-up chic)—and I was so taken with Diane Keaton's haircut on a cover of *Good Housekeeping* that I immediately had my hair guru copy it. The choppy layers looked fresh and modern, but I was warned that my hair didn't have the texture to pull it off. I refused to believe it. I left the salon excited about my new do, but my fine, straight hair soon drooped. As much as I tried, I couldn't replicate what the pro had accomplished, and ultimately the cut was too short for my round face. I was reminded, once again, that I am a low-maintenance gal when it comes to hair, and with my active lifestyle, I need to pull it off my face. It took eight months to grow it out, but I'm glad I gave it a go. We can't know if something is going to work or not unless we experiment. Now there are a host of websites where you can download your photograph and virtually try on different hairstyles and colors.

> Taaz.com is one of the many sites where you can upload your photograph to see how you look with different hairstyles and makeup colors. It helps take the guessing out of change. You can share these images online with your friends, or on Facebook, MySpace, or with Taaz's social network for the opinions of others.

W2W Closet Practice: Hair Truths

HAIRCUTS

A GREAT HAIRCUT IS LIKE GETTING A FACE-LIFT, BUT CHEAPER, QUICKER, AND HEALTHIER. Spend the money on a great stylist the first time around. It will be easier to replicate the cut for much less money once you know what works.

BEFORE CHANGING THE CUT OR COLORING OF YOUR HAIR, DISCUSS WITH YOUR STYLIST WHETHER THE DAILY UPKEEP OF YOUR NEW DO WILL BE LOW-MAINTENANCE, HIGH-MAINTENANCE, OR SOMEWHERE IN BETWEEN. If you find choreographing a brush and blow dryer a creative release or spending part of your day wearing rollers the norm, your options will be greater than for those who choose to keep it simple.

THERE ARE NO LONGER RULES ABOUT LONG HAIR and how it corresponds to age. It looks especially flattering if you are full-bodied, tall, or have a round face or weak chin. (Think Oprah, Susan Sarandon, me!) But long now looks best when its styled and shoulder-length or to the collarbone. Otherwise it can look limp, drag down your overall look, or appear that you are trying to hang on to the long hair of your youth, making you look older than you are.

SHORT HAIR CAN TAKE YEARS OFF YOUR FACE, especially if it's layered and styled. It is most flattering on petite women and those with defined chins or chiseled features. (Think Sharon Stone, Jamie Lee Curtis, Annie Lennox—spiky, choppy, edgy; Jane Fonda—layered, soft curls.)

WOMEN OVER FORTY ARE OFTEN ADVISED TO GET BANGS TO HIDE THEIR AGING FOREHEADS, but don't do it if your chin is not well defined or if you have jowls. It will only bring focus to those areas. Otherwise, unless your hair is curly, experiment with layered, side-swept bangs cut at an angle, so they can grow out easily. Bangs look best if you have a long, thin face. A bob with sharp bangs will give you a tailored look. (Think Katie Holmes, Anna Wintour, Eve Ensler.)

LAYERING GIVES HAIR AN OVERALL LIFT BY INCREASING ITS MOVEMENT. It softens features, especially when layers fall around your cheekbones. (Think Goldie Hawn.) Layering is also great for thinning hair, because it creates more depth in the overall shape of hair, and can prevent frizzy hair from taking on a pyramid look by distributing its fullness.

FOR A QUICK CHANGE, SWITCH YOUR PART. It often gives your hair a lift on top, as will an uneven part that zigzags, which also visually diminishes gray roots that grow in between colorings.

STAY AWAY FROM HELMET HAIR! It looks old and uptight. Hair should have movement and appear soft and less done, rather than stiff with age.

HAIR COLORING

WHY NOT? For a mid-life adventure, go for a new cut or completely change the color of your hair. Chemicals are getting gentler.

AS WE AGE, OUR COMPLEXION DULLS. Subtle highlights, just a few shades lighter than our natural hair color, will bring light and a lift to our face. (Think Meredith Vieira, Martha Stewart, Andrea Mitchell.)

DYING HAIR BLACK OVER GRAY WILL LOOK SEVERE. Again, lighten up black hair with highlights, perhaps with some caramel-honey colors near your face, or consider a white streak in front for drama.

TO GRAY OR NOT TO GRAY? EVERY GROWN-UP GIRL'S QUESTION. One of the soul-searching hair issues many of us grapple with is whether to color our hair to hide the gray.

Women who have prematurely grayed are likely to have a halo of silver-white hair that casts a beautiful light to their face. Others keep a shock of white hair in front as a foil to their dark hair for drama. But for most of us, our hair just grays in a dull way.

The benefits of remaining *au naturel* are obvious—less time and money spent on hair maintenance. But many of us are fraught with the anxiety of how we will be perceived by others, much less ourselves.

"I am not a vain person. I don't think I'll do my chin. After an illness when you have unwanted operations, it's hard to have more surgery. I am vain, though, about turning gray. I have the most beautiful fantastic fabulous friend who is letting her blond hair go gray and I tell her, 'You can't do that!' "

Julia, fifty-plus, art consultant, Richfield, Idaho

"After years of maintenance, I decided to let my hair do its thing. My hair is very thick and no professional seemed to get it right, so I started cutting it myself and got compliments on how it looked. But when the gray roots started showing, a close friend told me to start wearing a hat because men aren't attracted to women with gray hair. I took that to heart."

Jill, fifty, Long Island, New York

"I work in a youth-oriented environment, so I am very conscious and sensitive to perception, which is why I color my hair every four or five weeks, and give it a huge chemical beating twice a year to straighten it. I wish I could let it be natural and still compete effectively in business."

Lillian, sixty-plus, strategic sales and marketing consultant, Manhattan

"I held senior management positions at an early age. My hair started to gray in my twenties. I thought it would make me look more age-appropriate, so I let the gray show and haven't thought about it since. I now have thick silver hair and it has become a style signature for me. Women who have dark hair tend to go gray in a more flattering color than blondes—so we are lucky!"

Nina McLemore, fashion designer, Manhattan

"I want to look like a smart, sophisticated gray-haired woman, but the gray just makes me feel very tired. I don't dye it to look younger, but I have more energy as soon as it's out of my hair."

Goldie, sixty-plus, administrative assistant, Yonkers, New York

> "Is there a graceful way to grow old with gray hair? I asked my hairstylist if there was an elegant way to transition from color to *au naturel*—apparently I'm 75 percent gray. Shocked, she asked, 'Why would you want to look ten years older?' How silly of me, especially because my husband looks boyish and I didn't want to look older than him. Here I am eight years later with 'youthful' hair. *The au naturel* concept has its own I-want-to-be-me appeal and is obviously easier and less expensive to maintain, but it does age you and who really wants to add that to a vanishing waistline? I scour my budget for 'nonessential' items, but hair color remains steadfast! I think you have to have a lot of courage to take that step. I know a woman who I thought really pulled it off but she was advised more than once to dye it for job interviews."
>
> *Didi, fifty-five, Pasadena, California*

If you do decide to gray gracefully, spare yourself the long ordeal of growing in roots by cutting your hair short. An edgy cut can make all the difference between looking modern or dowdy. And if you need a mentor, look to Jamie Lee Curtis—the poster girl of our generation for going gray, and being proud of it. She shared her excitement in *More Magazine:* "Look at me! I've got gray hair and I don't care. I hate dyeing it—it's so boring and time-consuming. But it took me a long time to realize that and accept it."

Gray hair is a result of pigment loss—the less pigment, the whiter your hair. And because our hair is a sponge, it's important to use products especially designed for gray hair to shimmer and shine. Subtle highlights can add more depth and brighten the gray while removing any yellow cast.

Whatever color hair you choose to go with, it's important to take a fresh look at the colors of the clothes and jewelry you are wearing close to your face if you want to be seen in your best light.

Loss of Hair

Many of us are also dealing with thinning hair, which is often a result of stress, body health, or changing hormones, and should be discussed with your doctor.

One of my clients is a young mother who developed alopecia when she was pregnant. I give her clip-on extensions and work with her toupee to cover her bald spot.
—Edita Evon, Warren-Tricomi Salon, Greenwich, Connecticut

My hair gurus' advice is to take vitamins, see a dermatologist, and use products that are designed for thinning hair that will treat the scalp while creating volume. Adding color also thickens hair, but work with an expert who knows to avoid harsh chemicals.

Closet Confidential: Hair Crisis

"A few years ago, I had a hair crisis—my hair started thinning. I went to Philip Kingsley Salon for help, though I felt vanity personified when I saw a number of recognizable women there—among them an anchorwoman and a movie star. The consultant asked what vitamins and prescription drugs I was taking and gave me a long list of vitamin supplements, as well as some hair care products sensitive to hair loss. Since then I've discovered Nioxin's scalp treatment products, as well as Pureology shampoo and conditioner, which doesn't have any additives and is very gentle on the scalp."

Diane, sixty-four, design writer, Manhattan

Many of us have or will experience temporary hair loss as a result of chemotherapy. If you choose to wear a wig when undergoing treatment, have it styled by a professional.

"When your hair grows back, it's a different texture and sometimes a different color. One of my clients had straight hair, which grew back curly. It's important to have your hair styled as it grows back in, even if it's only one inch long, to keep it chic, trim, and shapely. You also must care for its health and stay away from harsh chemicals. Make sure you work with an expert knowledgeable about your condition."

Edita Evon, Warren-Tricomi Salon, Greenwich, Connecticut

Philip Kingsley is a leading expert on hair health and former chairman of the Institute of Trichology. Kate Winslet, Cher, Renée Zellweger, and Sigourney Weaver are just a few of the many who have had specific hair and scalp treatments created for them at Kingsley's Trichological Clinics in London and New York.

Hair Care

Think of your hair as a cashmere sweater. If you washed the sweater every day, it would break down the fibers. You don't want your scalp to dry and your hair to become dull by overcleansing. When you shampoo, concentrate on the scalp, not the ends, and treat it with sensitive products.
Jenny Cloke, Warren-Tricomi Salon, Greenwich, Connecticut

Products can rejuvenate hair by adding shine, volume, and bounce.

If your hair is dull, a tinted gloss will enrich its color. A moisturizing conditioner and a hair polish will liven dull, **dry hair.**

A hair masque puts **nutrients** into your hair.

For shine, use a clear henna or a gloss treatment. A hair polish will also **moisturize.** Thermal protecting sprays add shine and **flexibility.**

Flat and thinning hair can use a boost from products designed to add volume—shampoo, conditioner, spray, or mousse. Apply spray or mousse directly to the scalp, rather than distributing throughout the hair. Then bend over so hair falls away from your scalp, brush downward, and blow-dry. The heat and the angle will add volume.

If your hair is stringy, hair powder will absorb the oils, making it fluffier. Dab on loose translucent powder or a product designed specifically for this purpose (Bumble & Bumble Hair Powder).

Chlorine and well water adversely affect hair. The iron and mineral deposits build up in your hair, adversely changing its color while leaving it dull, limp, and full of static. Stay away from clarifying products. Most strip the good along with the bad. A salon professional can treat your hair back to health. Also consider replacing your showerhead with one that balances the pH and filters out contaminants (www.santeforhealth.com).

Caring Closet

The best brush for daily brushing is a natural-boar-and-nylon bristle brush. The nylon won't stretch or break hair, while boar bristles easily slide through hair, stimulating blood circulation in the scalp while distributing natural oils from the roots for shiny healthy hair.

If your hair is long and you decide to cut it short, consider donating it to **Locks of Love,** a nonprofit organization that provides hairpieces to financially disadvantaged children under the age of eighteen who have lost their hair due to an illness (www.locksoflove.org).

18

Finding Your New Colors

We dress to enhance our face from the shoulders up. It's the part of our body we most frequently critique in the mirror, and likely what we first examine in a photograph of ourselves. It's also the part of our body that holds our brain, the directress of our emotions, logic, and aesthetic judgments. Yet our daily dialogue with the mirror is slow to see how changes in the color, texture, and contour of our face and hair impact what we wear until the colors, necklines, and accessories that we counted on for years no longer *feel* as satisfying to wear. Worse, they might have become as unforgiving as the scrutinizing light we're subjected to in department store dressing rooms when trying on bathing suits.

> ### Closet Confidential: *Changing Colors*
>
> Laurie, fifty-three, pictured herself as a twenty-first-century Snow White—raven hair, pale skin, red lips. Professionals advised her to wear "winter" colors—those that are cool with more of a blue base rather than a warm, yellowish cast. She felt confident in her look until she started graying.
>
> When the few strands started to grow en masse, she darkened her hair until she saw a picture of herself taken at her son's college graduation. "I was shocked to see how harsh my hair made me look. I immediately went to my hairdresser and asked for blond highlights, and not to be subtle. Now I'm not really sure how I look. Are my colors no longer 'winter'? Do I need different clothes and makeup?"

Julie, a forty-something natural blonde with pale yet slightly ruddy skin, couldn't understand why she wasn't wearing her beautiful new beige suit that fit her perfectly—after all, it was an Armani. She couldn't articulate it, but she instinctively knew it wasn't flattering. When I encouraged her to try on other beige tones, she discovered that those with a lot more white than yellow in the mix gave her complexion a healthy, vibrant glow.

Similar to finding the right color of foundation for our face, there are a range of beige tones in fabrics—pinkish, yellowy, muddy, caramel-like, ivory. Their differences can ambush or enhance your complexion dramatically. Julie's beige suit had a yellow cast, which drained life from her face.

You Don't Need to Be a Color Expert to Reassess Your Colors

RECONNAISSANCE. Go through your closet and pull out those items you most frequently wear closest to your face. Take note. Is there a consistency to the color palette? The reason you enjoy wearing these clothes is that instinctively you know the color flatters your face.

EXPERIMENT. In varying light, hold up to your face clothes in various tones and colors. Don't hesitate to try on colors that you like, but thought you weren't supposed to wear. You may be surprised. One woman I talked to who is now silver-gray thought she could no longer wear gray clothes and was amazed to discover how they made her complexion look vibrant and her overall look very chic.

TRUST YOUR GUT. You will instinctively recognize how some colors make your face look pretty, while others make your skin look dull or harsh.

QUICK FIX. It's not realistic to throw out your existing wardrobe if some colors no longer flatter your face. You just need to wear them differently. Simply create a friendly buffer between your face and the offender—say, a colorful scarf or jacket. You can't go wrong wearing pearls or a white shirt to bring light to your face.

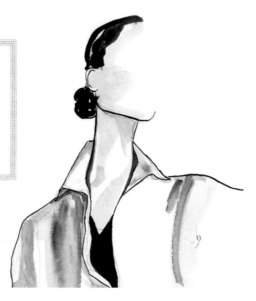

Closet Confidential: White Light

"I am always looking for perfectly fitted white long-sleeved T-shirts. Wearing white around the face makes an older face look younger and fresher. If it's well made, you can wear it under a dressy jacket or a simple sweater. It goes with everything. It doesn't matter who makes it, but pay attention to fit, and the finishing around the neckline. It's my best beauty secret."

Mary Louise, sixty-plus, painter, Portland, Maine

SEASONAL COLOR. If you are drawn to a color trend that doesn't flatter, wear it as an accent away from your face. Strategically placed, color can bring focus to or away from an area of your body. It can also give new life to your basics. Each season, fashion-savvy Becky updates the look of her black-and-white Closet Classics with a colorful new pair of mules and a sweater that she wraps around her shoulders.

COLOR MENTORS. With a watchful eye, we can be inspired to experiment with new colors by observing others. Oprah is a master at wearing colors that are vibrant and flattering. Hillary Clinton's colorful jackets and pant-suits cast a lovely light to her face while also setting her apart from a crowd. And sometimes it's simply someone admiring the colors we are wearing for the affirmation we need.

I see color better now that I've had laser surgery to correct my eyesight and to remove my cataracts. Now I am more adventurous in what I wear. When I get a compliment like "You look great in red," I'll buy red!
—Carmen, seventy-seven, world-famous model

LIGHTEN UP. As our features soften, wearing softer colors will flatter—pale pinks and blues, and varying tones of nude. Shades of purple—violets, plums, and periwinkle—are an antidote to sallow skin. And warm, sparkly colors that reflect light—gold, silver, bronze, and shades of orange with golden undertones—are energizing. White radiates light. Although black still works for some of us, other color classics—midnight blue, beige, gray, shades of brown—will appear less severe.

I was a brunette when I was younger. Now I am silver, so I wear light colors and black, of course. I don't look good in browns anymore. —Carmen, seventy-seven, world-famous model

SPARKLE. Pearls, gold, diamonds, or silver earrings and necklaces bring light to the face. The bolder the piece, the more light it will cast. Colorful stones like turquoise and amber can enhance the color of your eyes. High-maintenance Andrea wears huge gold hoops as her style signature. Blond-beige Julie was told by a style professional to only wear silver or white gold. After being coaxed to try on gold earrings, she was astonished at how much better they looked on her.

Rule of thumb: Gold jewelry looks best on blondes, redheads, and brunettes. Silver looks terrific on women with gray, platinum, or very dark hair. That said, experiment and be your own judge.

PICTURE-PERFECT. Turn up the collar of your shirt or jacket, wrap a scarf around your neck, or wear a bold necklace or earrings to frame your face with color. And remember that a monochromatic base in the rest of what you wear will not only help you appear taller and slimmer, but also make it easy to strategically place color close to your face.

illuminate
Oversized earrings are festive and bring attention to your face. Choose them in colors and finishes that cast a pretty light.

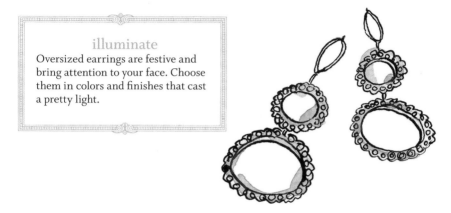

PRINTS. Some can look matronly after we're a certain age or visually overwhelm us, so wear them as an accent strategically placed—a little goes a long way. Animal prints and graphic patterns based on the classic geometrics (Tory Burch, Pucci) remain Closet Classics—they're sexy and energetic. Florals are feminine, but tricky. They look fresh on the young, but can make the rest of us look dowdy.

A change of color can also be a psychological boost. Jacqui from Bloomington, Minnesota, was forty-four when she was diagnosed with breast cancer. That's when she noticed a T-shirt that read PINK IS NOT JUST A COLOR, IT'S AN ATTITUDE. It inspired her to replace all her dark-colored clothes with those in pink. "I knew my husband wasn't going to give me the spending lecture, because I had cancer." She even painted her Harley-Davidson pink. Her message to the rest of us: "I love walking into a room with all you gals wearing black. It makes me look even brighter!" Clearly pink brings life to her face, and light to her heart.

Lilly Pulitzer

happy colors

Wearing happy colors makes us feel, well, happy, and not so uptight, which explains the continued success of Lilly Pulitzer, whose festive riot of colors and easy-to-wear designs have continued to thrive since they were first introduced to the Palm Beach crowd in 1959.

Eye color can be affected by the color of clothing, eyeglasses, or even a new hair color. "People perceive colors based on the light that bounces off objects, and some of that light—for instance, the red light from a red jacket—is going to be reflected in the eyes," says Dr. Norman Saffra, chairman of the ophthalmology department at the Maimonides Medical Center in Brooklyn. The change in color is more obvious in eyes that are light.

Closet Classics: Scarves

Scarves are decorative pieces of cloth that, depending on their size, can be worn around the neck, waist, head, or shoulders for starters. The closer to the face, the more impact a scarf has. An oblong shape in wool, fleece, or cashmere looks especially casual chic if you fold in two, drape it around your neck, then loop the ends through the folded middle. Scarves with ruffles or origami-like folds add dramatic flourish and distract from what lies beneath.

Wearing a classic silk headscarf around the neck with a pair of jeans is the perfect blend of cool and sophistication on any woman. Since the 1950s, Hermès silk scarves have been a paragon of style. First produced in the nineteenth century with woodblocks, then silk-screened with symmetrical equestrian imagery, the scarves take their luxurious sheen from the finish, which remains a house secret.

Closet Confidential: Wear It with Love

"[Breast] cancer is not the best or the worst thing that has happened to me. It's just another passage in life. Losing hair during chemotherapy, though, was very difficult. It's the anger part of cancer. I got a platinum wig, but I preferred wearing scarves—cloth or wool, because silk slides off. What was very special is that all my friends sent me scarves. I wore their friendship during that difficult time."

Julia, fifty-plus, art consultant, Richfield, Idaho

19

Pulling It Together

I knew I needed a look and got one. —*Maria Callas*

I think I have a sense of what looks good on me, but being able to put things together makes all the difference in the world, and that is my weak spot.
                    —*Valerie, fifty-two, entrepreneur, Bonita Springs, Florida*

Packing is my most favorite thing that I hate to do. It forces me to get into my closet and focus on what I need, what I enjoy wearing, and how to make it all work together. Pulling together the clothes and accessories in your Feel-Good Closet is like packing a suitcase for a great adventure—the adventure of your life. They fit, they flatter, but you might be uncertain how to coordinate them.

CLOSET CLASSICS. Having a "feel-good uniform"—those core basics that you can rely on to get through your life, or at least your day, comfortably and appropriately—will make dressing easier and more enjoyable, and shopping for clothes less overwhelming, because you'll have a better idea of what works for you and what doesn't.

COLOR CHIC. Limit the color palette of your Closet Classics. When I covered the Italian collections as a fashion editor, I was always struck (and inspired) by how chic Giorgio Armani looked when he took a bow after his show. Each season he wore his uniform—a navy tee or sweater and navy trousers in varying cuts and fabrics.

When your base is a solid neutral color or similar in tone:

- It gives you a long, clean silhouette.
- It's easier to add other colors and embellishments.
- It stretches your wardrobe, because you need fewer basic items to wear in varying ways.

To find the color of your Closet Classics, put the clothes you most *enjoy* wearing on your bed. Which neutral dominates—gray, navy, black, beige, white? If what you pull is colorful, what neutral do you usually wear to anchor them? That should be the base color of your Closet Classics.

KEEP IT SIMPLE. Closet Classics should have clean, classic lines. This will make it easier to add decorative or trendy pieces to the mix.

SHOP SMART. Over time, upgrade the quality, shape, and fit of your Closet Classics.

RECIPE FOR DOWDY TO DAZZLING: 3 PARTS SIMPLE + 1 PART CHIC. Leopard prints, ruffles, fiery colors, fun jewelry, attitude shoes, splashy clothes? What you wear with your Closet Classics is as unique as your facial expressions. It reflects your mood, your quirkiness, your preferences, your personality—your style. It's the fun part of dressing. I liken pulling it all together to roasting a chicken—get the basics down before adding the ingredients to reflect your particular taste or the season.

DON'T OVERDO IT. DECIDE ON A FOCAL POINT. Too much of a good thing will look like a mess.

Closet Confidential: Stylish Solutions

"I've learned to recognize that less is more. True simplicity is beautiful. When you have a few basics in black, white, and chocolate, it's easier to travel. It gives you the opportunity to pick up a few things along the way to add some fun to what you're wearing. So when I travel, I shop for things that are more original, thoughtful, and possibly conversational."

Sally, forty-six, environmental fund-raiser, Purchase, New York

"I dress myself much like I dress my home. My mother taught me to anchor a room by painting the baseboard a darker color than the room, which is what I consider the base of what I wear—my anchor. I start with a dark neutral base and then balance it with the fun of jewelry and shoes to punctuate my look."

Julia, fifty-plus, art consultant, Richfield, Idaho

"I try to wear one piece that is interesting because it is different. It took me a long time to figure out that different was good."

Beatriz, forty-nine, CEO of HispanAmérica and power yoga teacher, Newfoundland, Pennsylvania

"I don't buy a lot, but I do buy classic because I can't afford to change much each season. But each piece has something unusual about it—an oddity, usually in the cut. I almost always wear all-black with occasional accents of color—a colorful jacket or scarf. Black grounds the funny touches and eclectic shapes I like to wear, like harem pants, bold earrings, or something with an unexpected twist. I also like modern shoes and very high heels."

Andrea, fifty-plus, business executive, Manhattan

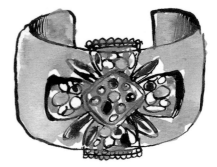

"I wouldn't define myself as a high-fashion dresser. My style is understated sophisticated, and comfort is important. I always wear a column of black that feel like pajamas (microfiber pants and scoop-neck top with a built-in bra that are machine washable), and always a colorful jacket, flat shoes because I have a bad back, and very bold jewelry. I have worn the same gold earrings for the last thirty years. When you develop a personal uniform, you feel confident. It's that feeling that you know you look great and appropriate when you put it on."

Lynne, sixty-plus, retail expert, Charleston, West Virginia

For me, I still gravitate to wearing white jeans or all-black. But I am much more conscious now of wearing a pretty color or decorative necklace near my face. And I'm always reaching for that one offbeat piece—an accessory or a clothing item—that makes me smile.

20

Shop Smart for the Rest of Your Life

When we change what we buy—and how we buy it—we'll change who we are. —Faith Popcorn

Win or lose, we go shopping after the election. —Imelda Marcos

I literally had a budget breakdown when my life was in transition. I was buying as though I was still in a financially secure marriage, working full-time in fashion, receiving a regular paycheck, and for a size 8 body.

I continued to justify my spending habits as I had throughout my career: It was expected of me to dress fashionably. This is not entirely untrue. Besides, I needed to clothe my new body. When the credit card debt began accumulating, I had a flash of the *Sex and the City* episode when Carrie Bradshaw realized that the cumulative cost of her designer shoes was the equivalent of the money she needed for a down payment on an apartment. I looked at all my great Closet Classics that no longer fit, and calculated the fortune I had spent on what I had considered investment dressing. If they had served me well for many years, I likened them to enjoying dividends from a stock investment. But I've since learned that stocks can vanish as quickly as a waistline.

My buying habits, like my closet, had lost touch with my reality. When we have a healthy relationship with our closet, we are constantly reassessing rather than remaining stuck in old patterns.

So how was I going to finance my new closet?

A lot differently than I had in the past.

Closet Confidential: *Money Matters*

"I have some things in my closet with tags still on. I am so embarrassed, especially now that I can't afford to shop anymore. I haven't even bought shoes in a year. I had more disposable income when I was twenty-two than I do now. Shopping was a sport to me. I would rationalize it, because I worked in retail, which often meant I paid less than 75 percent of the retail price. Now that I am in this new money situation, which is austere, I want to save for the rest of my life. When I feel the urge to shop, I stay away from pricey stores and designer boutiques and shop TJ Maxx. I also like consignment shops, but I am mostly selling to them now rather than buying."

gg, forty-plus, cosmetics entrepreneur, Rockport, Maine

We all shop for clothes whether we like to or not. Some of us consider it a treasure hunt, others a necessary chore. If it's an addiction, a quick emotional fix, or a drain on our credit cards, we and our closets will be filled with self-loathing.

There is no reason to give up on style whatever your size or budget. It's simply learning to Shop Smart. **Shopping smart is having the ability to discern how to buy the right stuff for your body, your budget, and your life.** It's not about owning a lot, but owning just what you need and enjoy wearing—those things that make up your Feel-Good Closet. No more, no less.

Closet Confidential: *Closet Awareness*

"I bought a lot of mistakes in my thirties. I used to feel secure with a closet filled with clothes. I would think I had nothing to wear and go through my closet and actually find clothes that I had forgotten about with the price tag still on. I guess it was part of the survival instinct: food, shelter, and clothing. Now I like a more orderly closet that isn't overfilled with clothes."

Jill, fifty, Long Island, New York

Always shop with your Shop Smart list. It will help you avoid shopping blunders as you get your closet in sync with your body and your life. Otherwise you may continue buying patterns that no longer suit you and become stuck with a closet filled with shopping mistakes.

Always know your budget, and then prioritize.

Closet Confidential: Budget Priorities

"I have always been frugal and resourceful because I was a student until my early thirties and had to budget my money. I think that's what I like about more creative resourceful dressing, but I also recognize the importance of quality. As my husband says, 'Quality will be remembered long after the price is forgotten.'"

Sally, forty-six, environmental fund-raiser, Purchase, New York

"I'd rather spend money on my home or traveling. I wear what I have over and over again. I feel like a New England dowager wearing clothes until they fray. How many black sweaters and black turtlenecks do I need? I used to have lots. Now I realize they were such a waste of money."

Jill, fifty, Long Island, New York

"I am hooked on bargain hunting online. It started as something to do when I couldn't sleep. Now betting against others in cyberspace auctions gives me the adrenaline rush others might get at a casino. I buy massive quantities of things I don't need, but never spend what I can't afford."

Lise, fifty-four, attorney, Providence, Rhode Island

"I usually don't tell my husband when I buy something because for the forty years before I married I never had to tell anyone. Besides, men don't get it. He can see how many black pants and shoes I have in my closet, so when I buy a new pair he doesn't understand. I try to explain there is black for each season and within that there is black for comfort, black for sexy, black for business, and then varying styles within each category. He knows I'm not extravagant and that I am not going to bankrupt him. Every time he makes a deal I don't say, 'Okay honey, I'm running to Bergdorf.'"

Susan, fifty-two, design entrepreneur, Manhattan

**Never shop when you are tired, depressed, stressed, bored, even slightly
intoxicated, feeling bad about yourself, or you can't sleep.** Buying with abandon is like having a blackout and waking up to a nasty hangover when the
bills come in.

Closet Confidential: *Retail Jeopardy*

"I am a random shopper, but I don't usually shop unless I'm on a long,
dull conference call. Then I shop online."

Ruth, fifty-two, attorney, Manhattan

"My soul has a mind of its own. Thank God, otherwise I would be
shopping on the Internet all the time!"

Susan, sixty, artist, Point Reyes, California

"I had a fender bender and felt so bad about it that I headed for the local
outlet mall and spent $147 on a blouse without trying it on. It was
European sizing. It never fit me. I never wore it. And now it sits in my
closet with all the other clothes that don't fit me. It was obsessive buying.
I realize now that I was punishing myself."

Lise, fifty-four, attorney, Providence, Rhode Island

Never shop with an enabler, especially one who has a larger shopping budget than you.

I spent an evening with a close friend who is an eBay addict. After dinner and sharing a bottle of champagne, she convinced me to bid on a pair
of cowboy boots—she has forty pairs and counting. I should have known
better, but I got swept up by the champagne and her coaxing (two no-nos).
I bought not one pair, but three! Granted, they were bargains, but I didn't
live in a cowboy-boot kind of world, at least not then, and I don't have the
closet space to house them all comfortably.

Always shop with someone whose style you trust if you're not confident in your shopping savvy. Working with a personal shopper (a complimentary service in many larger stores) or a knowledgeable sales professional can help you get out of a wardrobe rut by encouraging you to try on new ideas and stay away from bad ones.

> ### Closet Confidential: *Shopping Mentors*
>
> "I have found it best to shop alone or with a best guy friend (husbands included), but not with your best girlfriend or mother. There is an amazing amount of unspoken competition that is unintentional, but surfaces. I see it all the time, so think about who you're going to shop with before you head out."
>
> *Kay Unger, fashion designer*
>
> "My husband was bugging me to get some funky casual clothes, but I don't really know how to shop. I feel overwhelmed and lose my confidence when I do. I have a friend whose style I admire. I don't want to dress like her but like her cool look, so when I decided I wanted a fashion-forward purchase I asked her to help me shop."
>
> *Laurie, fifty-three, Westport, Connecticut*

As a working mother, I had little free time to shop, so when I needed something appropriate to wear to an afternoon Bar-Mitzvah, I made an appointment with the personal shopping service at Nordstrom. I described my coloring, height, style—classics with a twist—and my budget, which was comfortable with the sale rack. The sales gal pulled a range of choices that I would not have considered. Once I tried them on, I was delighted. They made me look like a more stylish version of me. I settled on a pale pink suit, and changed the gold-colored buttons to black jet, which was dressier and complemented the black patent heels I usually wore with suits. It was my favorite suit for the many years it fit.

Don't always buy out of habit. Refresh your closet by experimenting with different styles. Clothes look very different on your body than on the hanger. You'll know it works when you look in the mirror and smile.

Never buy into a trend just because it looks good on someone else or is considered "in" unless it looks good on you. Trust *your* gut. Otherwise you'll spend your hard-earned money on clothes that will just take up closet space or, worse, look silly on you.

Always refresh your wardrobe each season with at least one item that feels special to wear, looks good on you, and that gives your closet a boost.

> ### Closet Confidential: Update
>
> "I'm not a shopper, but if you don't shop for new things you'll start to look fuddy-duddy. If I need something like a party dress, I'll shop for it. Otherwise I concentrate on shopping to replace pants and other essentials when they get old and tired looking. And sometimes I'll just see something I like and pick it up."
>
> *Betsy, sixty-four, Ketchum, Idaho*

Always ask yourself, *Where am I going to wear this?* Sometimes we buy in to a fantasy that sits in our closet.

> ### Closet Confidential: Stuff of Dreams
>
> "I am no longer a big shopper, although I did make a buying mistake recently. I was feeling blue and to cheer myself up, I pictured myself looking very chic skiing in Vail so I bought these black furry boots that were pricey. I feel funny wearing them in the city where I live."
>
> *Jill, fifty, Long Island, New York*

Always try clothes on before buying unless you're willing to make the schlep to return them if they don't fit.

> ### Closet Confidential: Fit Fantasy
>
> "I often buy based on aesthetics—the fabric, color, texture, detailing—but without trying it on. If the size is too small, I try to convince myself that I'll fit into it one day. It's like art that sits in a box."
>
> *Lise, fifty-four, Providence, Rhode Island*

Never sacrifice comfort for style. They are not mutually exclusive. When you buy something that doesn't feel good to wear, you won't wear it very much. Your dollars aren't being well spent and your closet will become unnecessarily crowded.

Always buy for the body you have, not the one you wish you had. Choose fit over size. Sizing varies among manufacturers and designers. Snip out the tag if you're upset about the number. If you're between sizes, buy one up and have it tailored.

Always figure tailoring into your clothing budget. A tailor can give your clothes shape and proportion, making you look trimmer.

Always buy less, but buy better. Spend a little more on fabric, tailoring, and design. Spend less on trends.

Always give yourself time to shop and never settle. If you can't find *it* in one store, go to another. When you shop in a rush you'll likely settle for something that you aren't thrilled about, and consequently won't wear much.

Never buy if in doubt. Sleep on it. If you're still dreaming about *it* the next day, then it's passed the litmus test. Harvard psychology professor Daniel Gilbert, author of *Stumbling on Happiness,* explains that we quickly forget why something made us happy, which might help deter us from bad shopping habits—especially for those who shop as a form of therapy.

Always check out the return policy before purchasing anything. Know that boutiques often only give store credit for returns, so think twice or three times before you purchase.

Always save receipts and keep price tags on clothes until you wear them. Sometimes we fall in love with an item, only to find that we don't love it as much when it meets everything else in our closet. Same goes with mass-market cosmetics. They are 100 percent refundable if you don't like how they look on your face when you apply them at home.

Always treat your money and your closet with respect.

W2W Closet Journal: How Valuable Is Your Closet?

What kind of shopper are you?

_____

_____

What kind of shopper do you want to be?

_____

_____

How do you define value?

_____

_____

What are your spending priorities?

_____

_____

What are your saving priorities?

_____

_____

Are you honest about how you spend money or are you in a Ponzi scheme with your husband or credit cards?

_____

_____

Shop Smart: Chic on the Cheap

When I was a young girl, I remember my mother sewing upscale store labels like Bonwit Teller into bargain-basement treasures she found. Today, most women would deny they paid retail for a designer dress and would brag on about the great bag they picked up on sale at Wal-Mart.

No matter how good a deal is, never get swept up in the thrill of it all by buying more than you need. And don't buy anything you don't like just because it's on sale. A bargain is good only if you enjoy wearing and can afford it. Ask yourself if you would buy the same item if the sale price were retail.

Price haggling is not just for bazaars. Don't hesitate to contact a customer service rep for free shipping or look online for additional discounts. Phone calls are often more effective than online queries. Sometimes retailers are more accommodating if you use their store credit card or pay cash.

And for the many who express anger or frustration toward magazines that feature pricey clothes, consider them like paintings in a museum.

When we are exposed to quality and the zeitgeist of design, our eyes become trained to be more discerning when we shop for chic on the cheap.

Shop Smart: Mass-Market Designer Apparel

Great design is about inspiration, not imitation. Stay clear of designer knockoffs—besides being illegal, they'll cheapen your look. Today it's easier to find brilliant buys as designers bring their talent and eye for proportion, design, and interesting fabrics to all price points. Target, H&M, Wal-Mart, and Kohl's are but a few of the mass merchants who have successfully recruited high-end designers to create affordable stylish collections exclusively for them. These special offerings usually sell out quickly, so shop early in the season rather than waiting for sales.

Never sacrifice quality whatever the cost. Fabrics should look and feel luxe and not wrinkle easily. Those that have a bit of stretch blended with natural fibers are good bets. Stitching should be neat and not noticeable. Decorative details are a sign of value.

And just because it's cheap chic, don't hesitate to have it altered or tailored if necessary. Fit is a measure of quality. I picked up a long zebra-striped summer dress at H&M for under $40 and had it hemmed to my knees for $25 so I would wear it more frequently.

Shop Smart: Discount Designer Apparel

Stores like TJ Maxx, Daffy's, and Loehmann's, plus a host of online sites like Bluefly.com and Overstock.com, thrive on selling surplus designer clothes at slashed prices. These were the kind of places where my mother taught me the art of bargain shopping at a very young age. Each excursion was a treasure hunt. As we scavenged racks of clothing, I learned to distinguish the misses from those that could be transformed from fair to fabulous with a little altering, the addition of a missing belt, or a change of buttons. The clothes with labels that had been sliced were the gold standard. Superbly made in luxurious fabrics, they had once been for sale in swanky stores. My mother was convinced they hadn't sold because they might have been a little too jazzy or dramatic for most women, but to her they were winning finds. They added flair to her otherwise classic wardrobe. When you mix in a unique find with your wardrobe basics, you own the look. She knew no one else would be dressed quite like her.

Because merchandise is often displayed in a haphazard manner at these stores, take time to peruse the racks, then repeat. Visually we can be overwhelmed by the variety of offerings first time around. Today Loehmann's offers personal shoppers with a trained eye and merchandise savvy to help us troll for treasures.

Online shopping makes it easy to compare styles and prices, and like catalog shopping is a convenience for those who don't have access to a variety of merchandise or the time to get out and shop during store hours. Some sites are by subscription and will send you e-mail alerts for designer sales.

Many designers and retailers offer merchandise online that they don't carry in stores because of limited floor space. This is especially true if you're shopping for petite and plus sizes. J.Crew sells a full selection of bridal party attire exclusively online.

Always check the return policy. On some sites, it's unforgiving. If you're not sure about sizing, shop sites where returns are easy and order a few sizes until you become familiar with a particular brand. It will cost you in shipping, but may ultimately be worth the savings. Don't be afraid to haggle for free shipping. You'll have better success if you communicate with a service representative on the phone rather than online.

Most online retailers offer discount coupon codes. Search online for sites dedicated to sharing this information.

Shop Smart: Designer Sample Sales

At the end of each season, designers have showroom sample sales. Runway pieces are sized to fit models. There is a better variety of sizes when designers sell end-of-season merchandise from their stores.

New York is the hub for sample sales because it is the heart of the fashion business, but there are sample sales in cities that have their own garment district or regional design showrooms like Los Angeles, Chicago, and Atlanta. LazarShopping.com is a good resource for listings.

Shop Smart: Discount Malls

Discount malls are also a favorite destination to buy branded clothes for less, but unless it is a small design house like Etro, much of the merchandise is specifically created for these outlets. They may not be quite the caliber of design that you had anticipated.

Shop Smart: Retail

If you frequent certain retail stores, make contact with a personal shopper or a salesperson in the departments you favor. Ask them to alert you to the arrival of clothes you might like, as well as upcoming sales.

When retail stores advertise upcoming sales, scope them out a few days in advance. Often a salesperson will hold items if you put them on a credit card.

If you purchase anything retail and it goes on sale within fourteen days of purchase or if you find the item for less elsewhere, many retailers will refund you the difference if you've kept the receipt.

You can often find interesting buys for less in the men's department (sweaters) or teen department (accessories, petite-size clothing).

Shop Smart: Consignment and Thrift Shops

Closet Confidential: *Treasure Trove*

"My daughter recently commented, 'Older women look best in really expensive clothes.' I now buy all of my clothes at high-end resale shops. For the first time in my life, my closet is bulging with fabulous designer clothes—Armani, Jil Sander, Brunello Cucinelli. I feel like a million dollars when I put these things on, and because they're resale, they cost not one dime more (and often way less) than the more mass-market brands I had been wearing. I look for timeless, classic cuts and perfect fit. And I don't wait until I have a fashion emergency to shop. I sometimes have things for months before the occasion arises to wear them, but when it does, boy, am I ever ready!"

Marilyn, sixty-plus, Internet entrepreneur, Chatham, New York

The best consignment and thrift shops are in upscale neighborhoods, because that's where the very fashionable and very rich unload their fabulous designer clothes.

Thrift shops are often affiliated with a charity, whereby donors get a tax credit. Consignment shops are run as a business—sale proceeds are split between the shop and donor.

Thrift shops are less discerning than consignment shops in what they accept, so merchandise is generally marked at lower prices.

You can locate consignment and thrift stores in the Yellow Pages or by going online, but you need to visit them to determine those that complement your style and standards. My youngest daughter got hooked on Ina in Soho, New York, after learning that it sold all the slightly worn clothes featured in the television series *Sex and the City,* whereas I have found a cache of way-reduced Hermès scarves and bags at a Roundabout consignment store in Greenwich, Connecticut. And note there are specialized consignment stores: those for bridal gowns, plus-size clothing, furs, formal wear, jewelry, maternity, children's clothes, and more.

Although thrift and consignment shops have end-of-the-season sales, shop frequently as things come and go quickly.

When you shop with an open mind, you can pick up items that will distinguish your look. If you stumble across a find, scoop it up. You won't regret it. We make our biggest buying mistakes when we shop under the pressure of time. I bought a priceless magenta Chanel jacket adorned with jet beading and the signature gold-chain-lined inside hem at a tony thrift shop in Indianapolis for less than the cost of two pedicures. When I'm traveling somewhere upscale, I shop these venues for real finds.

Really smart shopping means buying things that will have a long life in your Feel-Good Closet. Recycling what we no longer wear or buying at thrift stores, consignment shops, backyard sales, community fairs, or online sites such as Craigslist, eBay, or various barter sites keeps stuff in circulation rather than in landfill. A law of reciprocity—one person's junk is another's gems. Knowing someone else will benefit from what we no longer wear makes it easier to dejunk our closets. Shopping at local stores is also a way of supporting your community.

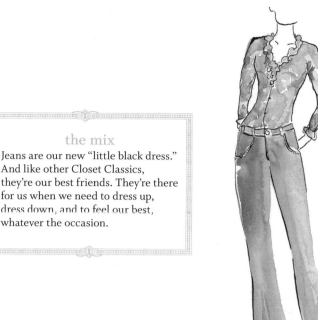

W2W Closet Practice: The Mix

Great style does not have to be expensive. It's all about confidence and the mix—real with faux, high fashion with street chic, inexpensive with not so inexpensive, simple with decorative, sporty with dressy, artisan with mass-produced, classic with whimsy.

Sharon Stone rocked the fashion world when she wore a Valentino skirt and Gap top as a nominee and presenter at the Academy Awards in 1996. "My friend Ellen [DeGeneres] suggested I go into my closet and get out five of my favorite pieces . . . [I wore] a Valentino ready-to-wear skirt, an Armani dress worn as a coat, and a Gap T-shirt . . . I thought, 'A Gap T-shirt to the Oscars? Hey, I'm nominated [for *Casino*], and I'm presenting two Oscars, so why not have some attitude?'"

A departure from former first ladies, Michelle Obama dresses as stylishly in affordable off-the-rack clothing as she does in high-end designer wear, and she doesn't hesitate to mix the two.

Stylish women don't need to wear high-ticket items to feel confident or comfortable. If it's in our Feel-Good Closet, why not mix things up? It's how we choose to mix that creates our unique personal style.

bejeweled

Faux is fabulous even on your feet. Bejeweled sandals add lots of wow to the simplest of summer Closet Classics.

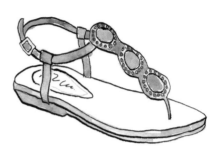

Closet Confidential: Tricks of the Trade

"As a young underpaid magazine editor, I had a limited clothing budget and learned to substitute designer clothes with knockoffs then mix them in with the real thing. Later when I worked at *Town & Country* magazine I learned the importance of accessories in polishing a look. If I was in Chamonix or Aspen writing a story on new ski schools and fabulous après-ski spots, or when interviewing fashionable people in fashionable places, I always wore one thing that was winning. If I couldn't afford a new snowsuit, I would upgrade my goggles or ski gloves. It was better to finish an outfit however inexpensive it might be with an Hermès scarf, a cashmere shawl, or a fabulous piece of jewelry that was real or chic faux by Kenny Lane. It would make everything else I wore look stylish."

Kathryn, sixty-five, writer, Manhattan

"Kal Ruttenstein (legendary retail guru who was the fashion director of Bloomingdale's for three decades until his death in 2005) told me that the key to being well dressed is to buy an expensive well-fitting jacket and you can pair anything with it—jeans, a $24.99 skirt, et cetera."

gg, forty-plus, cosmetics entrepreneur, Rockport, Maine

Kenneth Joy Lane's fabulous faux jewelry has been a favorite of royalty, first ladies, celebrities, socialites, and fashionable women since it was introduced by Saks Fifth Avenue in the 1960s. He created Barbara Bush's signature three-strand faux pearl necklace, and it's speculated that the Duchess of Windsor is buried wearing a jeweled belt he created for her. His jewelry is available in various museum stores, specialty stores, on QVC, and exclusive pieces are sold through Avon representatives. His vintage pieces are considered collectibles selling at major auction houses.

"You don't need to have a lot of money to have good taste. You just need to invest in a few key basics to present your best self to the world. I have some really good jewelry from my husband and family. I have fun wearing it with street jewelry. If it has good bones, it doesn't matter how much something costs. That's why my Outsider Art and my formal Georgian furniture look good together in my home."

Julia, fifty-plus, art consultant, Richfield, Idaho

Shop Smart: Best Buys on a Budget

Jeans. Designer labels aren't necessary for great style. Levi's—what miners wore in the gold rush—have a long history of cool. Wranglers have a story of being the jeans cowboys wear, perhaps because they have a tight fit and are inexpensive. Cowgirls like them because they are cut to flatter the derriere. Black, white, and blue are basics that can be dressed up or down.

White shirts. Don't spend too much money because they yellow with time.

Sweaters and shirts found in the men's and boys' departments are often higher in quality and lower in price than those found in the women's department.

Head-to-toe basics in black. Black is elegant, slimming, goes with all other colors including navy blue (think French gendarmes), and is forgiving of flaws in quality and in our own perceived body flaws.

Casual summer dresses, when simply designed in colorful cotton.

T-shirts in solid colors with a bit of stretch for shape and with sleeves in varying lengths.

Active wear offers a range of comfortable fabrics, good fit, and great styles. It can be mixed with dressier closet clothes.

Shoes. Summer sandals, ballet flats, and colorful trendy pumps don't need a designer blessing to look chic and stylish. They need to fit comfortably.

Hosiery. Brands like Hanes offer consistent quality, which is why designers trust them to create their branded lines.

Faux jewelry. Don't be shy about it: The bigger the better.

Art jewelry. Shop museum shops.

Street boutique accessories. Great finds, but stay away from designer knockoffs!

Reading glasses. They don't need to be high-end prescription lenses to do the job; over-the-counter works for most of us. When the price is right, you can build a wardrobe of options.

Bags. Those made from recycled materials have good karma. Summer canvas, straw totes, and those in teen departments and mass-market stores offer fun designs at even more fun prices.

Ethnic clothing. Shop in Chinese, Indian, and other ethnic neighborhoods for authentic designs at budget prices.

Mass-market brands that have staying power are cool chic: Timex, Hanes, and Levi's jeans are among those that deliver value and style.

Shop Smart: Sustainable Chic

sus·tain·a·ble (sə-stā′nə-bəl) adj.
Capable of being continued with minimal long-term effect on the environment.

When my youngest daughter was five, she came home from a day at camp with her legs covered in mosquito bites. Before she went to camp again, I sprayed them with insect repellent. A few hours later, I got a call that she'd had a seizure and was in an ambulance racing to the hospital. Tests and tests and tests later suggested poisoning from DEET, a potent ingredient in many bug sprays. I had never heard of this chemical. I simply bought a well-advertised bug spray. Now I read labels carefully for toxic ingredients.

As a mother, I also became concerned about the presence of hormones in dairy products and pesticides in apple juice. Despite the extra cost, I switched to organic dairy products and juices.

My awareness of the connection between the environment and our health intensified when my mother was first diagnosed with breast cancer. She lives in an area of Long Island that has a high incidence of the disease. That's when I started buying bottled water. Then one of my younger sisters was also diagnosed with breast cancer. She lives on the West Coast in another cancer hot spot. These diagnoses were the first cancer in our family for generations and suggested environmental factors. I now try to shop for organic or fresh local foods. As food writer Michael Pollan advises, "Don't buy anything to eat that contains an ingredient your grandmother never heard of."

After I developed asthma as a grown-up, I discovered that a perfume I had been wearing as my signature scent is particularly harmful to lungs. I became more cognizant of the everyday chemicals I put on my body and of the toxins that may be polluting the air in my home. I have switched to buying more eco-friendly cleaning and beauty products.

What I wear has always impacted how I feel; yet now I am becoming aware of how it impacts the earth and the people on it. Knowing that it takes one-third pound of pesticides and fertilizers to grow enough cotton for a single T-shirt that is not organic doesn't make me feel very good about buying conventional cotton anymore. I don't want to compromise on quality and design, but I do want to live in harmony with the world.

Al Gore suggests in the educational exposé *An Inconvenient Truth* that people often need to be broadsided before they rethink the choices they make in how they live. His own father stopped growing tobacco only after his sister died from lung cancer. After seeing the movie with my ten-year-old nephew Max, he commented, "I wish I didn't know about all this, but I'm kind of glad I do, so maybe I can make a difference."

Thankfully, many in the fashion industry share these concerns. **Several designers and manufacturers have launched a tireless quest to create desirable and stylish clothes in eco-fabulous materials.** Bamboo has been transformed into luxurious lingerie, candy wrappers have been recycled into hip bags, and machine-washable cork clothes have made their debut on the runways in Paris.

Large manufacturers like Levi's and Wal-Mart are integrating organic cottons into their private-label products. Katharine Hamnett, Britain's first lady of fashion, teamed with Tesco, a British supermarket chain, to design a full line of organic clothing. She's already launched Katharine E. Hamnett (*E* for "ethical" and "environmental")—a pesticide-free sportswear line. Several other high-end designers including Stella McCartney (who has a line of organic skin care products), Giorgio Armani, and Eileen Fisher are experimenting with designing clothes in a variety of eco-friendly fibers. Bamboo is softer and more breathable than cotton; it's fast drying, it's moisture wicking, and it inherently prevents the growth of bacteria, keeping us odor-free—perfect for active living and the changing climates of menopause. Nontoxic Tencel, a wood derivative, drapes beautifully. Hemp is strong, silky, and hypoallergenic. And there is a growing demand for wool sheared from sheep given organic feed, without the additives to which our skin and lungs are sensitive. Purists like Of the Earth are cutting-edge in their use of sustainable fibers, whereas others might blend them with synthetics for a better fit. Do your research.

Several companies have gone to the next step in their socially conscious efforts by scrupulously monitoring the manufacturing process for fair-trade practices. Edun Apparel, founded by Ali Hewson, her husband Bono, and designer Rogan Gregory, is committed to bringing long-term sustainable employment by manufacturing their radically chic garments in developing countries. Their mission is to "deliver the fishing rod rather than the fish." Other groups like Alabama Chanin combine ecologically conscious materials with the artisan craftsmanship of local women.

But unlike the food industry, the fashion industry doesn't yet have strict guidelines to make it easy for the consumer to choose between conventional and organic. Los Angeles–based designer Linda Loudermilk, a self-described earth warrior, creates a 100 percent earth-friendly and 1000 percent sexy luxury line of clothing—the ultimate in eco-glam. She hopes her "luxury-eco" will become a universal code to further consumer awareness.

All these efforts are reshaping eco-fashion from tree-hugger green to eco-chic. These are not just trends in a trendy business; they're an evolution. The times they are a-changing. We have reached a tipping point in that what and how much we consume can be considered vulgar rather than rights for bragging. The status shopping bag has been replaced in stature with recycled reusable bags to hold our groceries as well as fancies.

Conscious consumerism is not just about what we buy, but how we discard. Patagonia, affectionately called Pata-Gucci by wilderness guides for its stylish and pricey active wear, has long taken the lead making eco-conscious decisions in the materials used in its active wear. The firm has also placed drop boxes in various stores so we can easily drop off Polarfleece we no longer wear for recycling. Nike also has drop boxes for worn-out sneakers they will transform into basketball courts in underprivileged neighborhoods. The Polo Ralph Lauren Foundation rounded up thousands of used jeans and converted them into even more thousands of square feet of environmentally friendly insulation, which in conjunction with Habitat for Humanity was used to rebuild homes in places of need.

Admittedly, I'm not yet in the habit of seeking eco-friendly garments. And I am not suggesting a radical overhaul of our closets, but an awareness of the choices we make when we shop. I subscribe to the Aborigine words: *The more you know, the less you need.* If it's a question of cost, buy less, but buy smarter. Buy local when possible. Smart buying decisions don't end at the checkout counter. Recycle clothes rather than discard or neglect them. Choose friendlier ways of caring for them. Switch to a dry cleaner who has converted to nontoxic solvents—which coincidentally put more fluff into wools, add brilliance to silks, and aren't as harmful to the life of clothes, not to mention our lives.

Perhaps it will be our children who will come to expect eco-chic as a natural option in their choices of what to wear and how to live. Meantime we can teach them by example to be better stewards of the planet. That to me is living a life of truly great style.

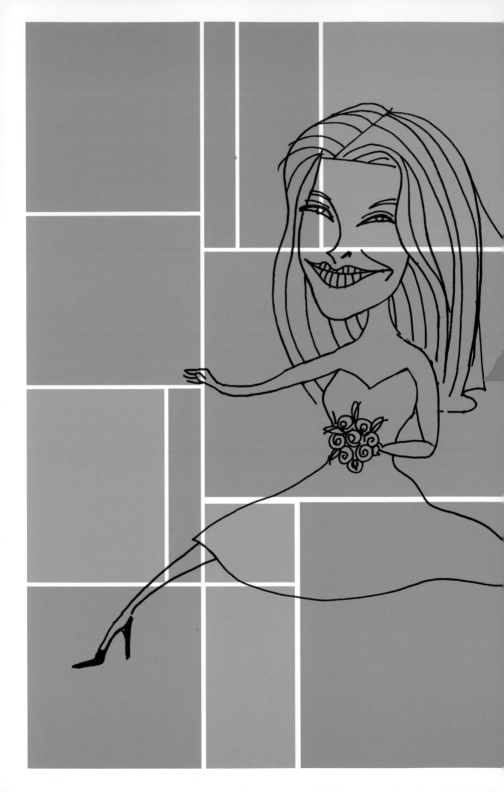

I was so much
older then,
I'm younger
than that
now.
—Bob Dylan

PART FOUR

CLOTHES MEET LIFE

I am not
a has been.
I am a will be.
—Lauren Bacall

21

Strategies for a Working Closet

What to wear can fill us with trepidation on any occasion, especially one burdened by expectations. The emotional connection between what we wear and how we feel is especially powerful as we dress for the many clothes-meet-life situations unique to this next part of our lives. Some will be planned, some unexpected. Many will be joyous; others will call upon all our resources to cope. It may mean figuring out what to wear when interviewing for our next career or for a younger boss, going to a class reunion, dealing with the hot swings of menopause, becoming the mother of the bride or an encore bride. When we get it right—a balance of what we want our clothes to communicate and how we want to feel wearing them—what we wear will provide a feeling of comfort, protection, and confidence when we need it most.

Okay, just one more time: **When you are clothes-confident, you will feel more body-confident, which will help you feel more life-confident.**

I'm 8 years older, 10 pounds heavier, and a half-inch shorter, just in time for HD television.
—Kathy Lee Gifford joking about returning to morning TV to host the fourth hour of NBC's *Today* show

My youngest daughter just graduated from college. Her first interview is today for what might be the job that begins her career. She has spent days preparing, researching the company and its competitors. She asked me to shop with her for an interview outfit. She settled on a gray knee-length skirt, white tailored shirt, and fitted gray jacket. She found a black leather tote large enough to hold a red folder that contains her resume, business cards, and notebook. "I want to appear organized and not have to rummage through my purse." The hunt for simple closed-toe black pumps was unsuccessful. Most heels had open toes and hovered at four inches high—"I love these shoes but they make me look like a sexy secretary"— or they were shiny. She'll borrow mine. She thinks it's important to connect with the interviewer personally, perhaps with a colorful bag or shoes that have more personality, but she'll save that to wear on the second interview. Meantime, she's decided to tie a pretty scarf around the handle of the tote to add some color.

As my daughter finds her way, many of us, too, are trying to reinvent our look once again. She will look to her boss and savvy colleagues for guidelines, but it's likely we are discovering that what's appropriate for us has become more complicated.

Some of us find Style Mentors by observing women in power, politics, and on the news. Lynne, a fashion retail consultant in Charleston, West Virginia, notes: "Professional and high-profile women in the community want to look appropriate, confident, and powerful. Many look at Michelle Obama and Nancy Pelosi as style mentors. Obama's sheath dresses and Pelosi's Armani and St. John suits are pretty but also project power and confidence. These women know a no-no in the boardroom is to dress in a manner that has their male colleagues speculating on how fast they can get them into bed."

Many of us may be starting a new career of sorts. Don't kid yourself: Retirement becomes a vocation. To quote Gloria Steinem, "What would I retire from? Life?" Or perhaps we find ourselves working in a younger environment, maybe even for a younger boss.

Kathie, fifty-two, and Holly, forty-nine, run workshops where 85 percent of the women who attend are under thirty-five. "We have wisdom to share, but worry, 'How can someone their age relate to me?'" Kathie and Holly recognize the importance of dressing for their audience and want to update their look without appearing trendy.

What we wear is a form of communication. Professionally, we need to dress in a manner that reflects the business we represent and how we want to be perceived within that community. Thankfully, we're no longer afraid to dress like women. If we're required to wear a uniform, it may simply be our choice of earrings that differentiates us from the pack. According to the *Wall Street Journal*, even female construction workers are starting to wear hand-painted hard hats and pink tool belts to show their *I am woman!* pride of succeeding in a traditionally male occupation.

As we get older and the competitive job market becomes younger, **what we wear must become increasingly strategic as a means to distinguish ourselves with confidence.** Even if you don't have a younger boss, the chances increase every day that you will. It's your job to adapt, not theirs. Our Feel-Good Closet must be as versatile, intelligent, prepared, appropriate, and current as we are.

Strategy 1. Communicate

When I started my business, I became doubly aware of the impact my wardrobe had on a presentation. It's part of the sales pitch, because it's the first thing a client sees. As an interior designer, I am selling my services, my expertise, my taste, and myself. The hardest part is to figure out the style statement you want to make. I want my clothes to say

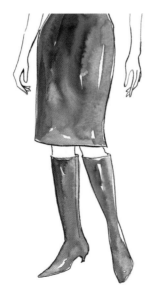

great gams
Boots worn with opaque and patterned tights are a modern way to dress your legs, unless you work at a very conservative firm where sheer hosiery is required.

"classic, tailored, creative, professional" while projecting ease, confidence, and enjoyment.
—Elaine, forty-four, interior designer and author, Manhattan

Essentially, you are the brand, and what you wear is the packaging. As with most brands, packaging needs refreshing over time to remain competitive and relevant. Like Elaine, identify your brand strategy.

Strategy 2. Distinguish Yourself

As a trial lawyer it's important to get and maintain people's attention. I'm essentially a salesperson. I dress to get noticed and be different, but not disrespectfully. A line I walk, just like women did when they started wearing pants when only skirts were permitted. When I was younger I was conflicted on how to achieve this because I have always been a nonconformist, but now I pair tailored items with colorful shawls or interesting jewelry and my personal signature— cowboy boots. I recently tried a case wearing a different pair each day. The jury was enthralled.
—Lise, fifty-four, attorney, Providence, Rhode Island

Lise's confident approach to what she wears in the courtroom comes thanks to her years of experience in trial law and to her unwavering sense of self. She successfully differentiates herself from the status quo without being inappropriate. The jury takes notice.

Strategy 3. Look Contemporary

A senior vice president in advertising, fifty-year-old Sallie straddles corporate and client meetings while directing a younger staff. "I need to look contemporary in a field that demands it," she says, "while not looking foolish. By incorporating one trendy piece among an otherwise classic wardrobe I avoid being arrested by the fashion police."

Sallie's winning strategy combines classics (authoritative, ageless) with edge (creative, current).

Strategy 4. Project Confidence

Everyone was younger in the office where I worked, even the owners, so I decided to distinguish myself. They wore jeans so I dressed up. I wore power suits with trend items—a leopard-print shirt, great shoes and bags. I entered meetings looking in charge. When you dress with confidence, you project it.

—Karen, fifty-plus, event planner and former vice president of sales and merchandising for an apparel manufacturer

When we met, Karen had just come from teaching a merchandising class at a design college. She looked modern and feminine in clothes she's owned for years. A sheer ruffled lavender blouse worn under a brown fitted sweater softened her look, while a black techno-fiber skirt was a modern classic. She completed the look with a flourish of long and short necklaces.

Strategy 5. Be Relevant

Lillian, sixty-plus, a pro in strategic marketing, dresses more casually for younger clients. "It sends a message that I'm flexible—not set in my ways. I won't wear jeans or a pin-striped suit. I opt for relaxed knits and bold jewelry. In corporate meetings, I'm very tailored but add color with a jacket or accessories."

When I met with Lillian, she was about to meet with publishing executives wearing cream-colored trousers, a simple black blouse, bold ivory-and-black bangles, and zebra-print shoes.

Strategy 6. Adapt

Forty-five-year-old Kathy, an interior designer in San Francisco, says: "I dress the same for everyone, but I stick closer to the classics when dressing for older clientele. With younger clients, I wear my skirts a little shorter, shoes a little hipper, and trendier jewelry."

Kathy had a busy workday ending with a cocktail party. She wore a three-stranded (faux) pearl necklace, cashmere sweater, houndstooth pencil skirt, black tights, and leather boots with sexy-yet-sensible heels.

Strategy 7. Project Your Personality

Unlike when I was young, I now resist blending in. I didn't want to conform then, but I had to in order to succeed. My father was black and my mother Latin, which makes me Blatina? My father pressured me to dress like the white culture to fit in, yet stand out with my intelligence. Black men can pull off that straitlaced look, but black women can't. Besides, my Latin roots gave me a love of color and patterns, but women in managerial positions when I started working dressed so uptight. I loosened up when I became more successful and when yoga crept into my life. It inspired me to give up my suits and to stay away from wearing black.
　　　　　—Beatriz, forty-nine, CEO of HispanAmérica and
　　　　　power yoga teacher, Newfoundland, Pennsylvania

Beatriz's style evolution is emblematic of women in the workforce. Gone are the days when we had to wear mini men-suits with girl ties, skirts, and hosiery, and when wearing pants was verboten. As we succeeded professionally, we became more confident dressing to express our professional savvy.

Strategy 8. Be Open to New Ideas

After thirteen years in corporate, Judy moved from Wisconsin to the beaches of Mexico and went into sales, reporting to younger managers. "The transition challenged my Midwest power suits. My closet is becoming hipper. I now meet with fashion executives wearing Lucky jeans. I was a sales kitten in my twenties, had the classic older-sister look in my thirties, and now I'm the hip sales matriarch. This was my best reinvention ever."

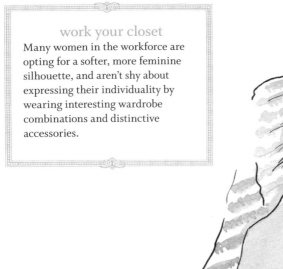
Strategy 9. Refresh

It's unflattering to compete with twenty-something-year-olds; besides, I don't want to look like anyone else. I prefer pretty sweaters to corporate jackets. My jewelry is a mix of classic and contemporary, which sets me apart from younger and older women.
     —Hilary, forty-five, magazine executive, Westport, Connecticut

By mixing the old and the new in her closet, Hilary communicates experience while being open to fresh new ideas on the job. It reflects her unique style, which she has honed over the years.

Strategy 10. Determine Your Uniform

Hillary Clinton was one of the first highly visible women in politics to wear pantsuits. They became her working uniform. When she won her senatorial bid she joked, "Sixty-two counties, sixteen months, three debates, two opponents and six black pantsuits later . . ." Hillary personalized them with colorful tops, scarves, and jewelry. For her reelection speech to the Senate, she wore a jacket in her favorite color yellow, which tapped into her inner girl.

When she was on the campaign trail seeking the Democratic nomination for president, her suits became more colorful. When she graciously relinquished her bid in support of Barack Obama, she once again acknowledged her functional wardrobe when addressing her constituency of female supporters at the Democratic convention. "Thank you to my sisterhood of traveling pantsuits," she said wearing a tangerine-colored pantsuit.

Hillary appears comfortable and confident in her functional and appropriate wardrobe of pantsuits. They allow her to focus on her work and not worry about what she is wearing.

These women are aware of why they wear what they wear. They are in constant communication with their closet and the world they are engaged in. Over time each has successfully refined her message with a working closet of unique classics and accessories. The way they put it all together is how they adapt while distinguishing themselves to succeed and survive.

What I Wore to Sell This Book and Why

When my agent told me she had scheduled us to meet with several publishers who were interested in this book, I knew that what I wore was crucial. I had to appear confident in my expertise as a style authority and as a woman negotiating this next part of her life. I wanted my clothes to say, *Kim knows her stuff, and women can relate to her. She can inspire and empower them to manage their body, budget, life, and closet transitions with élan.* After all, that was the message I was selling, and the next stage of my career was hinging on it.

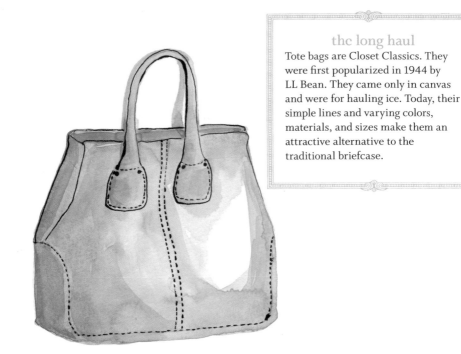

Since the Alien landed and my business had evolved from working in an office to writing wherever I happen to be, I had been working my closet with every bit of professional know-how I have. My life had become infinitely more casual than it had been for decades, and the ease of the everyday clothes that dominated my Feel-Good Closet now were too *laissez-faire* for these meetings. Nor did I want to spend money on an interview outfit. This was the start of a long journey in redefining my self-image, not a quick fix. I wanted what I wore to be an authentic part of the story I was sharing—the continuing dialogue among my closet, my body, my budget, my life, and me.

It was a warm Indian summer in New York City, and the zeitgeist remained summer-casual. I needed clothes for three days of interviews. I literally spent hours trying on combinations of tops and bottoms until I got it right. Finding pants or a skirt that fit was challenging. Body shapers were imperative. Strategically positioning the splash of dash was paramount.

OUTFITS 1 AND 2. Basic black pull-on pants were a good, easy start. Next came a black jacket that I had long since been unable to button, but it continued to give me shape and said *professional*. (I don't believe that blacks have to match.) I wanted to add some pizzazz—that's the style factor. I alternated wearing a wildly patterned Pucci shirt that would say *stylish classic*, and a white blouse with a flurry of cascading ruffles in front, which was one of those timeless blouses that also happened to be in vogue. Each would add personality to my basics while detracting from the Alien, but there was no way I would take the jacket off because I had to squeeze into these shirts, causing unsightly back flab. I was candid about the situation when I had hot flashes during several of the interviews. Why not? I wasn't trying to pretend that real life doesn't intrude on what we wear; I was addressing how to deal with it when it does.

The black Manolo Blahnik sling-backs that I had bought many years before when I needed comfortable pumps for my ailing feet—and was in a fashion industry entitlement frame of mind considering my finances—continued to say *quality, success, timeless, chic*. The bright green suede tote that my daughter Carolyn persuaded me to buy, precisely because it wasn't black like almost everything else in my closet, was functional and cheery. I finished the look with my signature jewelry—a large black wood ring, gold hoop earrings, and an oversize heart-shaped crystal necklace made by my friend Kazuko.

OUTFIT 3. Tailored cotton khaki-colored trousers that had enough stretch to allow me to zip up. I wanted to wear something more interesting on top, so I chose a sleeveless black origami-styled confection. It had become one of my favorite summer basics because it was modern and stylishly distracted from the Alien, so I am having it copied in other colors. I pinned on a colorful brooch and exchanged the green tote for one in basic black.

OUTFIT 4. Those Feel-Good Closet pieces got me through three days of interviews feeling comfortable and confident. Then a rogue meeting popped up later in the week, and what I had been wearing was dirty. I had no other appropriate pants to wear that even remotely fit, so I rifled through my skirts. I decided on one in black leather that would give me a stylish edge even if I couldn't zip it up. Next, I tried on every black light-weight knit I owned—most appeared to have shrunk around my midriff and in length. I placed those traitors into a recycle bag for my daughters and sisters to enjoy. I found one tucked away that I had previously considered dowdy because of its unshapeliness, but now was just what I needed. I wore it with a large faux pearl necklace and a white cardigan that I wrapped around my neck to brighten up the overall look and draw the eye upward away from my middle. My legs are in good shape but uneven in color, so I wore black textured hosiery to bring the eye downward away from my middle, and tempered the look with conservative black pumps.

I made it through the interviews feeling good about what I was selling and about how what I wore backed me up. It takes time and patience to pull a look together while you and your closet are in transition. But a closet challenge is also a way of rediscovering the closet classics you can count on, even if they need to be refreshed over time. Our accessories become increasingly invaluable for style expression, to draw attention to our assets, and to boost our mood and confidence.

The good news for me, and I hope you will agree, is that I sold this book. And here we are.

W2W Closet Practice: Work Your Closet

My partner at Chic Simple, Jeff Stone, and I were asked to give a presentation on value and style to the top global leaders at the Ford Motor Company. I held up to them a black sheath dress I had taken from my closet and explained that Coco Chanel first created the little black dress in the 1920s, a time when black was only worn by shopgirls and for those in mourning. *Vogue* compared it to the Model T, because it was affordable style available to all women. It remains a Closet Classic more than a century later.

I then held up to the dress a variety of accessories and asked the executives what Ford car each "woman" was driving. Pearls and pumps? A Lincoln. Colorful bag, sweater wrapped over the shoulders, fun flats, big hoop earrings? Thunderbird. Jean jacket, fishnet stockings, boots? Mustang. You get the idea.

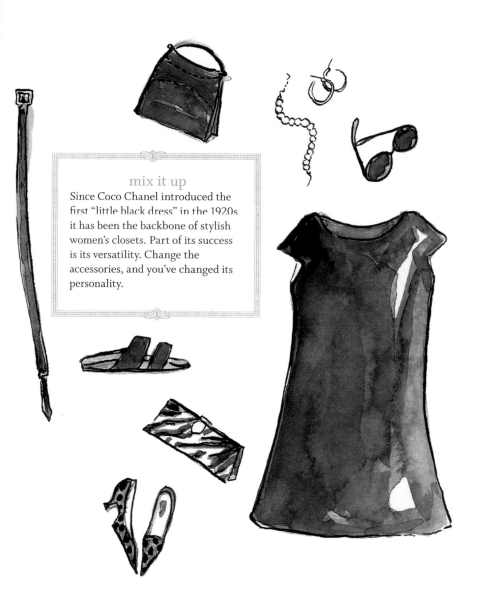

This practice will help you visualize your personal style message while getting you out of a wardrobe rut. Take your Closet Classics and rework each with other wardrobe items and accessories for a variety of looks.

22

Re-Dressing Your Sexuality

All women want to *feel* pretty.

Since the first time we slipped on a fig leaf, we gals have been aware that how we dress is an expression of our sexuality. It may be with the utmost modesty, or as a blatant means of seduction, or somewhere in between, but it is always with the intent of *feeling* pretty. It's validation that we are connecting with the world and to ourselves as women. None of us want to feel as though we have disappeared.

Closet Confidential: *Invisible Me*

"I used to be the hip mom and sexy wife until recently. Clothes had always helped me move through my day with confidence and assurance. Now at forty-five I feel like I am drifting aimlessly down the aging trail and no longer know what to wear."

Penny, fund-raiser for American Diabetes Association, Tucson, Arizona

"I first noticed that men weren't looking at me any longer as a desirable woman when I was forty and still in good shape. I now understand why wealthy women get boy toys."

Ruth, sixty-plus, designer, Manhattan

Throughout our lives, our sexual identity tries on a lot of different emotional and physical shapes depending on our age, the situation, and how we feel about ourselves. Sometimes we equate our femininity with being sexual. Other times we may feel more sensual. And there may be moments when we wonder, *Where has it gone?*

How we dress to connect with our sexuality is an expression of how we define ourselves as women. It's our declaration to ourselves that we are still vital, whether we're going through menopause, mourning the loss of a spouse, becoming a bride or the mother of the bride, dating again, challenged by an illness, becoming an empty-nester, or simply wanting to be noticed as a woman. When we're in transition, we can become confused. But if we give up on ourselves or allow ourselves to be defined by others, we disappear.

Closet Confidential: Defining Moments

"When my elderly mother was in the hospital dying of cancer, she asked me to help her put on her jewelry and lipstick every day. She told me that it helped her feel like a woman."

Scott, fifty-five, attorney, Scranton, Pennsylvania

"There's a DA I work with who was so incredibly beautiful that at first I found it intimidating—long blond hair, very fitted suits, leggy, and wore what we call 'Staten Island' red pumps. Her husband encouraged her to wear short skirts and tight clothes and would buy her Victoria's Secret underwear. Then she had a baby and completely gave up on her appearance. I told her not to be a cliché, but to be a hot mama. Just because you become a wife and mother doesn't mean you're still not you. She hasn't listened."

Ruth, forty-two, attorney, Manhattan

"When I turned fifty, a special person came into my life and told me how beautiful I was. I couldn't believe it at my age, but that comment changed my outlook and the way I dress. I gave away all my clothes that dragged me down, and replaced them with those that gave me back my femininity, starting with lingerie. What I wear now flatters my figure instead of hiding it, and makes me feel like a woman."

Suzette, bartender and cleaning service owner, Henrico, Virginia

---

The desire to *feel* attractive can motivate us to dress with thought or paralyze us into retreat. There are many, though, who avoid the gym because they no longer feel good about their appearance. Marylyn, a sixty-year-old retiree in Boise, Idaho, goes to the gym at the times when the older ladies exercise so she can feel good about herself in comparison. In contrast, her husband goes when the young guys work out for motivation—a Mars and Venus thing? I studiously avert my eyes from the mirror when exercising—why kill the buzz with an unnecessary reality check? And I am sure to wear all-black workout clothes to visually diminish the bulges and a fun pair of earrings for girlie cheer. I also get ideas from other gals of what to wear and what not to wear.

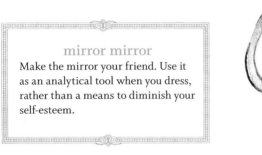

mirror mirror
Make the mirror your friend. Use it as an analytical tool when you dress, rather than a means to diminish your self-esteem.

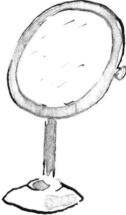

Dressing the Inner Girl

We face mirrors in life that force our inner girl to confront our outer girl—class reunions, seeing ex-beaus, blind dates, becoming the mother of the bride or a grandparent. These occasions are a measure of time that can challenge our "girl confidence" if we allow it.

The mother's face was of a fading prettiness that would soon be patted with broken veins: her expression was both tranquil and aware in a pleasant way. However, one's eye moved on quickly to her daughter, who had magic in her pink palms and her cheeks lit to a lovely flame, like the thrilling flush of children after their cold baths in the evening.

—Tender Is the Night, F. Scott Fitzgerald

When I'm with my daughters (twenty-one and twenty-five) I am aware that men's eyes often move in haste from me to appraise my daughters. It reminds me how men of all ages used to flatter me with their attention. I don't feel threatened by the course of evolution. It makes me rethink the woman I am at this time in my life. Over time, it's natural to give up a degree of narcissism. The torch may have passed, but it doesn't mean the flame isn't being stoked.

Closet Confidential: *Rules of Attraction*

"When I go to the beauty salon, I see all those young cute gals wearing those tight little tops and fitted jeans. I tell them to appreciate it while it lasts, because one day they'll be my age and won't be able to dress that way anymore. I mean I'm not dead. I notice attractive men, but I can't dress to attract like that anymore."

Carolyn, sixty-two, grandmother, Boise, Idaho

Why not? Carolyn is right not to dress in a saucy manner, but she can dress to *feel* attractive—which is ultimately what attracts.

One happily married gal I interviewed knew she was going to run into her first serious boyfriend at a party. She hadn't seen him in many years. "Seeing the ex-boyfriend—that is another category altogether—it contradicts anything and everything I said about not trying too hard. All of a sudden, methods such as injections, surgery, or anything else that's legally available and makes you look better seems totally reasonable. It also means engaging a clothing stylist, hairstylist, skin specialist, hair colorist, and makeup artist so that I look completely natural. Let's face it, who's kidding who? There are just some people in your life that make all the wisdom and sensible ideas you think you've acquired completely fall apart."

In some ways a blind date is easier than seeing an ex or going to a class reunion. They have no visual history of you. They see you in the now. Since the Alien arrived, I have been avoiding the annual lunch I usually have with my very first boyfriend. Before seeing him again I needed to regain the confidence that disappeared when I lost the girl and her closet that I felt defined me. These situations give us pause to reassess what *feel-*

ing pretty means to us now. If we're smart about it, we get in front of the mirror and into our closets to get out of a rut and kick butt—our butt.

Sexy Closet

sex · y [sek-see]
—adjective, sex · i · er, sex · i · est.
1. concerned predominantly or excessively with sex; risqué: *a sexy novel.*
2. sexually interesting or exciting; *radiating sexuality: the sexiest professor on campus.*
3. excitingly appealing; glamorous: *a sexy new car.*

> *I need a young, young man to drive my middle age blues*
> *When you reach middle age, you don't want a final chapter*
> "Middle-Aged Blues Boogie," Saffire

A friend's mother moved into an assisted living community after she was widowed in her late seventies. There was a gentleman there whom many of the gals found very attractive. When he singled out one for a kiss, the others grew jealous and wondered, *Why not me?* My octogenarian mother doesn't want to leave her home unless she's carried out in a coffin, but when I told her this story of flirtation and other stories of sex and romance in senior communities, she became intrigued. Not that she's in any hurry to explore this venue for meeting men. Since my father died decades ago, she's been in a long-term relationship with a beau that keeps her quite preoccupied.

Sexy—sex, intimacy, companionship, flirtations—doesn't have an age limit. Philanthropist Brooke Astor was a legendary flirt well into her nineties. She smote men of all ages, while women of all ages admired her skill. *Cougars*—the term coined for women who date much younger men—are becoming more common in the public eye. Actress Demi Moore was forty-two and actor Ashton Kutcher twenty-seven when they married. Kim Cattrall, who played the cougar Samantha in *Sex and the City,* has a much younger beau offscreen, too. She told Oprah, "I'm limitless as far as age is concerned . . . as long as he has a driver's license." Ivana Trump, The Donald's first wife, whose fourth marriage is to a man twenty-four years her junior, has been quoted as saying, "I prefer to be a babysitter than a nursemaid." Online dating sites for singles over fifty are thriving. And in a survey conducted by the AARP, single women over forty-five who are dating want companionship, but don't necessarily want to remarry. As Katharine Hepburn said, "I'll get married when I decide to give up the admiration of many men for the criticism of one."

Married or not, many women over fifty are jump-starting their libido with sex toys and vaginal lubricants for their own pleasure and to deal with the Viagra-popping men in their beds. (That's one closet I don't want my daughters to rummage through.) *Use it or lose it* takes commitment.

Sexy conjures up all sorts of visions unique to each of us. Some of us feel we are. Some of us don't. Some feel we were. Some of us wish we were now. Others couldn't care less. Whether we define ourselves as sexy or not, how we choose to clothe our sexuality evolves with time. And those changes should be reflected in our closet.

Closet Confidential: *Fetching Fancies*

"I think about what sexy looks like more and more. I don't want to appear frumpy or tarty. A nice décolleté can be very sexy. I am buying more V-neck tops—even in T-shirts. They have a softer, prettier look to them. If I'm wearing something low-cut, I'll layer it under a shawl, sweater, or jacket. Stilettos aren't for me now as comfort is most important, but a nice heel is sexy. I also think long hair is sexy and elegant, especially when it's pulled up loosely. I used to only wear my hair up when I exercised until my husband told me how much he liked it swept up. Initially I thought, *I've blown my hair dry, why would I put it up?* but now I find it sexy, too."

Susan, fifty-two, design entrepreneur, Manhattan

"I haven't lost my spark, but dressing sexy to me now is all about sensuality. When I wear a four-ply cashmere sweater and my husband rests his head on my shoulder, well, one thing can lead to another."

Bev, sixty, food writer, Chicago

"I've never dressed 'sexy.' I'm not comfortable with it. Whenever I've tried, I've felt foolish. Wearing really, really expensive clothes like Armani and Gucci that are exquisitely tailored in incredible fabrics make me *feel* sensual. A lot of it has to do with the quality of the fabric. I also wear sexy underwear. A friend took me to Kiki De Montparnasse in Soho. It was quite an education. What I bought was a Valentine's gift for my husband (of twenty years) and for me."

Sally, forty-six, environmental fund-raiser, Purchase, New York

"I have cleavage and think it's a good way for me to stay sexy, but the sexiest and most versatile accessory I own is a silver fox boa. It might not be politically correct, but it's really a boon to my wardrobe. I wear it over jackets and a slim black reefer coat. A beautiful jacket that's shapely but not too tight and in an interesting fabric like silk damask, taffeta, brocade, bejeweled, or sequin-sprinkled covers up a multitude of figure imperfections and looks sexy and feminine. A pretty black or white cashmere sweater worn over well-cut trousers and some signature personal jewelry is sexy anytime, almost anywhere."

Kathryn, sixty-five, writer, Manhattan

"For me sexy is showing a little cleavage and wearing tight jeans! After I lost the weight (it's been five years since I lost 137 pounds), I rewarded myself with breast implants. For the first time in my life, I actually have a shape! Other than losing the weight, it was the best thing I had ever done for myself. I feel so pretty!"

Brenda, fifty, executive assistant, health care, Frisco, Texas

"It's been so long since I've felt sexy, much less dressed sexy! If I had the assignment to dress sexy tonight, I don't know what I'd put on. Relying on cleavage is too much of a joke these days. I think sensual is the new sexy for me. I'd make sure that every milliliter of my skin was hair-free and soft. I'd find a scent to wear that made me feel delicious and therefore project deliciousness. I'd treat myself to manicure, pedicure, maybe a facial. In short I'd put the emphasis on feeling ultra-sensual and projecting that."

Didi, fifty-five, Pasadena, California

"I think women start to look more masculine after they're fifty-five, especially if they're on their own. I don't want to look like a superwoman. I want to be perceived as a gentle, mature older woman who still looks good, has dignity, and is treated in a respectful manner, so men feel comfortable asking to assist me with their masculine strength even if I don't really need it. So I think it's important to wear little feminine touches—earrings, a pearl necklace or a pretty brooch, a sweater with ruffles and tops in muted colors—dusty rose, cornflower blue, cornstalk yellow—especially when wearing pants."

Goldie, sixty, administrative assistant, Yonkers, New York

"I like mystery. Dressing sexy to me means hinting just a little— revealing collarbones, the upper back. I have a sheath dress with a high side slit that feels sexy to wear."

Beatriz, forty-nine, CEO of HispanAmérica and power yoga teacher, Newfoundland, Pennsylvania

"I like sexy, but not crazy sexy. To men, sexy dressing usually means cleavage. Recently when I wore a low-cut dress and a pearl necklace, a funny, flirty man I know told me, with his eyes fixed on my breasts, what lovely pearls I was wearing."

Diane, sixty-four, design writer, Manhattan

"I just can't do the overtly obviously sexy thing. No pumps and negligees for me, unless it's a joke. I personally feel sexiest when I'm at my fighting weight. That's really the key for me. Then anything I put on feels sexy, whether it's flannel pajamas or a snug sweater."

Leah, fifty-plus, writer, San Miguel de Allende, Mexico

In 2006, Match.com reported that people over fifty make up the site's fastest-growing segment—a 300 percent increase since 2000. Some sites, like PrimeSingles.net, cater specifically to the over-fifty crowd.

Dressing Sexy—but Not Necessarily for Sex

I never thought I'd spend ninety minutes with my closet before a blind date figuring out what to wear. Quite honestly, before my divorce, I never thought I'd be on a blind date again.

This was not my idea. I have never had any flirting skills. My philosophy has always been that by doing things I enjoy, I would meet people with common interests (and perhaps "the" guy) along the way. My friend Judith was impatient with my lack of progress and was on a mission to move things along.

She met him at a book party. He was recently separated and tried to pick her up. Judith was flattered but married. Rather than blow him off, to my horror, she arranged for us to meet. After a few get-to-know-you e-mails, we arranged to have dinner together. I have since learned that sharing a meal rather than a drink is brave (actually, stupid) for a first meet, but neither of us was skilled in the art of blind dating.

What should I wear? What do women wear on blind dates? What do I want my clothes to say about me? Who am I anyway? What do men find attractive in a woman? The emotional inner dialogue about dressing for this date surprised even me.

As online dating services have grown to be efficient matchmakers, many women advise dating as much as possible, because it feels awkward at first sitting across from a complete stranger and brushing up on the art of pleasant conversation, especially if you've been in a long-term relationship.

Some women dress to let the guy know that she has expensive taste, so he knows what he might be getting into. Others prefer to keep it casual, but still attractive: their best-fitting jeans, a top that subtly shows off an asset (cleavage, waist, shoulders), great shoes, and light on the makeup and jewelry.

Closet Confidential: Date Your Closet

"I dress for myself, not to attract someone. I like the comfort of pants, but if I like the guy and he behaves, for a second date I'll wear a skirt and high heels. Men love that. I recently went on a date with someone who told me how attractive I was and how much more attractive I would be if I lost ten pounds. That was it for me. He keeps calling, but I won't see him again. I can look in the mirror and be critical, but I'm my own sentinel. I don't want anyone else to do that."

Andrea, fifty-plus, business executive, Manhattan

"I was in my late forties when I divorced. Some of the first things I bought to wear were nice underwear, a fur coat (the furrier couldn't believe how silly women of our generation were to buy our own fur coat rather than have a man buy it for us), pretty robes, glamorous ski clothes, and cocktail clothes. I was starting to date."

Kathryn, sixty-five, writer, Manhattan

"I've been a widow for several years now, and have since been out on a number of dates, many of which were arranged online. I learned that understated is the way to go. It gets down to choosing classic pieces from my closet and adding an accessory or two. One of my 'uniforms' for casual dates is a jean skirt with a funky woven wide leather belt, black tights, suede flats, turtleneck sweater worn under a close-fitting down vest, and a fun scarf. I keep the jewelry to a minimum—usually silver bracelets and studs. The guys are all about it."

Tessa, fifty-five, personal trainer, Wayne, Pennsylvania

What I wore. It was a warm summer evening. I decided to wear something more feminine than pants, but not too girlie. My black stretch cotton sleeveless dress was relaxed yet sophisticated (*she's stylish but not high-maintenance*). I could wear it with the low-slung beaded belt I had recently bought in Machu Picchu (*not that we would discuss my belt, but wearing it made me feel adventurous and worldly*). The dress showed off my arms and legs (*she's fit*), but I needed to wear my strapless bra with it, which makes me look much bustier than I am (*false packaging!*). What if the relationship escalated? Would he be surprised, disappointed, annoyed at this deceit?

I went back into my closet. I had professional clothes, workout clothes, very dressy clothes, but what did I consider dating clothes? Ultimately I decided to dress for my own pleasure and went with the black dress and illusion-making bra.

It turned out to be a fun evening. There was the promise of many more to follow. Of course when people connect, it doesn't matter what they're wearing, but that night my clothes gave me confidence. It was also another one of those clothes-meet-life moments when I needed to take a fresh look at what my closet was saying about me. It had become complacent over the years of a long marriage. I now needed a dating closet!

Dressing to Please

When we dress for someone special, we anticipate what they might like to see us in, or we know from their previous comments. What we wear is partially determined by culture and geography. If we live in a community where women wear provocative clothes, we are apt to be influenced by this. If the community is conservative, we will likely dress in a more reserved manner.

Closet Confidential: *Guys and Gals*

"I dress for myself or for other women. My husband never comments."
Hilary, forty-five, magazine executive, Westport, Connecticut

"When my husband asked me to wear something sexy to a dinner we were having with friends, I was confused. What did he mean by sexy? Unlike some women I know, I had never thought about buying sexy clothes. I always just wore what I liked, but I wanted to please him. I look good when I bare my arms and shoulders so I wore a clingy black top that showed some cleavage and bared one shoulder with fitted jeans, dangly earrings, and killer shoes. He liked the way I looked, which made me feel sexy."

Karen, fifty-plus, event planner, Westchester, New York

"Now that our daughter is a little older, my husband and I have more private time to have a date night together. I'm not a sexy person, but I brush my hair, put on some lipstick, and make sure my shirt is clean before he comes home at night. I make an effort."

Theresa, forty-six, political volunteer, Manhattan

"I dress for myself and for my husband when we go out together. I know what he likes and what he doesn't, but I don't buy specifically for him. It's about choosing what to wear from what I have. He likes color and doesn't find black appealing, so I look for color in my closet. I will also wear some of the great art jewelry he has given me over the years."

Susan, fifty-something, mother of four young children and former Manhattan advertising executive, West Marin, California

"I don't dress for men, I dress for me."

Carmen, seventy-seven, world-famous model

W2W Closet Practice:
Make a Date with Your Closet

- Rate your closet's sex appeal.
- Sexy is a state of mind. If showing some cleavage feels sexy to you, play it up with a great bra. A semi-sheer top with a camisole underneath is subtly suggestive, as is baring shoulders.
- Wear fabrics that *feel* luxurious against your skin such as cashmere, silk, and soft cotton, or clothes with decorative embellishments, like lace, ruffles, something sparkly or in a pattern or color that is dressier than you would simply wear every day.
- A dress is a feminine alternative to separates. A high slit in a long skirt is suggestive, as are flounces.
- Shoes with toe cleavage are sexy.
- Hosiery is sexy. The sheerer, the sexier. Patterned hosiery is also sexy.
- Decorate yourself with a bit of bling.

Also, pay attention to your hair—try wearing it in a softer, more feminine way. Give yourself a manicure, pedicure, shave, or wax. Dab on some perfume that's headier than your everyday fragrance.

The Boudoir

Whether it's the destination for romance or where you two just sleep, why not dress with allure some nights to make the evening a bit more special?

- A long and luxurious robe is more suggestive than revealing.
- A full slip is sexy innocence because it's practical yet provocative—think Elizabeth Taylor in *BUtterfield 8,* Faye Dunaway in *Bonnie and Clyde,* Reese Witherspoon in *Walk the Line.*
- Baby-doll lingerie discreetly covers our middle while being fun and flirty.
- A corset with garters and stockings is porn-star sexy.

I have learned during the course of writing this book how to dress to detract from the Alien, but the sexy lingerie that fills my Divorce Closet hasn't been getting much wear since my middle expanded. The lacy thongs with matching bras no longer give me body-confidence. I need to take a fresh look at my Sexy Closet.

W2W Closet Journal: Rendezvous with Your Closet

What do you feel sexy or sensuous wearing?

23

Jewelry from the Heart

I have never felt more emotionally or physically naked than when I removed my wedding bands. For more than twenty-one years they were emblematic of my identity. Everything else in my life had changed since I first started wearing them—my family, my homes, my jobs, my friends, my interests, my closets—but those two rings, and what they represented, were a constant. They grounded me. Without them I felt uncertain. Did I appear as different to the world as I did to myself? Even my hands looked unfamiliar to me—lonely.

Closet Confidential: *Precious Gems*

"After I was widowed, I had my wedding band cut to fit my pinkie finger. I will never take it off, even if I remarry."

Tessa, fifty-five, personal trainer, Wayne, Pennsylvania

"After my divorce, I sold my engagement ring to the diamond mart. Holding on to it would have been a reminder of failure."

Jill, fifty, Long Island, New York

> "I wear my engagement ring on my right hand now. It isn't typical—my husband designed it. I guess if I were with someone who was bothered by me remembering my deceased husband this way, I would take it off. Otherwise I don't think I will unless our daughter eventually wants it."
>
> *Aimee, fifty-five, San Francisco*

For some, jewelry is a form of status—married, engaged—a trophy of self-worth. For others, it's a form of self-expression or fashion—art jewelry and fabulous faux are as desirable as any gem, and the bolder or more individual the jewelry the better, to reflect the women they have become.

> *Closet Confidential: Inspired*
>
> "I celebrated my fiftieth birthday in Paris where I noticed a woman wearing a spray of jeweled insects on her shoulder. It incited a passion for researching and collecting whimsical costume jewelry with pedigree. Wearing these conversation pieces has since become my personal signature."
>
> *Teresa, fifty-seven, social worker, Manhattan*

Many women have started buying their own "serious" jewelry rather than waiting to be given pieces by others for special occasions.

> *Closet Confidential: Another First*
>
> "I bought a sapphire ring with my 'divorce' money. Every time I wear it I feel empowered, sort of like when I first bought myself a car."
>
> *Roni, forty-nine, executive assistant, Fishers, Indiana*

I had a similar transition. The spiritual me connects with the bold crystal heart-shaped necklace that I have worn almost every day since my divorce. It has become my signature piece. The fun me enjoys wearing oversize amusing rings in plastic, wood, and other nonprecious materials. The practical me values my classics—pearl necklace, black pearl earrings, large gold hoops, diamond studs, and Cartier tank watch. Each holds a treasured memory.

I have moved on with my life, but continue to save my engagement ring and wedding band. They are my personal artifacts. If I had a son, I would consider it bad luck for him to offer the engagement ring from a marriage that ended to someone he wanted to share an eternity with. But I have daughters. I lost one diamond from a set of diamond studs given to me when my eldest was born. I am considering using the engagement diamond to replace the other half of the lost set. Just like marriage—a union may be broken but reconstructed with love. I think that would be a fitting wedding gift for one of my girls.

For me, I'm not waiting around for him—whomever he may be—to get it right. I don't hesitate to buy my own jewelry to celebrate the most special of occasions—me!

Closet Classics: Jewelry

Aside from any personal *sturm und drang,* there is a practicality to wearing jewelry. Watches tell time. Pearls and gold bring light to our face. Bold necklaces detract from aging necks. Aged hands are less noticeable when eyes are focused on an oversize ring—real or faux. Wearing the jewelry you own in different ways—mixing old and new, real and faux—is what personal style is all about.

24

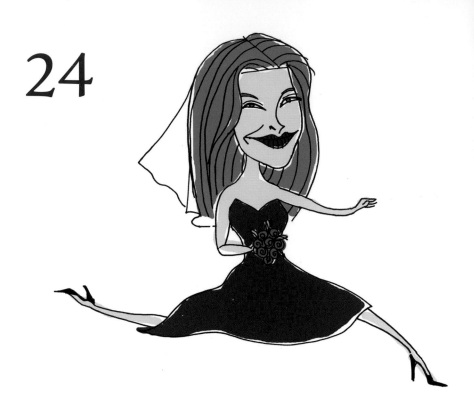

I Do, I Did, I Do

I am a romantic. I believe in love and I believe in living happily ever after. If it's with a Prince Charming, then why not rejoice—long white dress and all? When I share this thought, friends are quick to remind me that I bought in to that fantasy the first time around, and besides we all know that marrying a prince doesn't guarantee a happy ending. As my sister Jill remarked, "Women today should get married in business suits. At the very least, you can wear them again." Perhaps she's right, but I like to think it would be worn over a sexy cami and a fabulous pair of shoes.

So what are we supposed to wear if we give it another go or first marry at an age when we no longer blush? Even etiquette books acknowledge there are no steadfast rules, although veils and orange blossoms remain no-nos. In reality, nowadays anything goes. Naturally what we wear should reflect the time of day, the setting, and our personal style.

I still envision my friend Jane's wedding number three in a very elegant Park Avenue apartment. She wore a tea-length champagne-colored satin charmeuse dress cut on the bias and held one perfect calla lily. She and the setting were the height of elegance. It inspired me to imagine how I would do it all over again long before that was even a remote possibility. Even happily married women fantasize about what they would wear if they were to remarry—to the same man, of course.

Closet Confidential: What If?

"In my imagination, I would wear an off-white cashmere full-length turtleneck dress to show off my hard-won and newly found body. We'd stand in front of a roaring fire at home and entertain witnesses in some version of how we normally entertain. This isn't Queen for a Day—you've been through that fantasy trip. This time a little solid ground underfoot seems more apropos."

Marilyn, sixty-plus, Internet entrepreneur, Chatham, New York

---

Many practiced brides favor wearing pastel colors, but blushing brides no longer have the exclusive on wearing white—a color that once represented purity in Western cultures, mourning in Eastern. White is now considered a symbol of joy.

When Michele, sixty-five, and her longtime beau married, there were no attendants except a granddaughter who wanted to be a flower girl, and a grandson who got roped into being a ring bearer; he carried the ring on his teddy. The bride wore white silky trousers and a sparkly white jacket. A friend remarked, "Pants for a bride? Not for me, but come to think of it, Michele always wears pants. So *c'est juste.*"

My favorite wedding dress satori was when a colleague mentioned she might remarry in a tangerine-colored dress that she had fallen in love with. Wow! I had never considered the possibility of wearing a color so daring for the occasion, but aren't we all daring to give it another go? I recently saw a photo of a bride who wore gold. That, too, struck a chord—she dazzled in the delight that she had finally struck the jackpot.

Most importantly, what you wear should be a reflection of how you want to feel. Betty Halbreich, author and legendary personal shopper at Bergdorf Goodman, told me that almost every woman who comes to her wants a dress and jacket for the occasion, but leaves with something more sensuous or what she calls "grown-up sexy." Questions like length and whether to cover arms depends on how it looks—there are no rules.

Closet Confidential: Dressing for Next

"I wanted to rejoice in my sexuality the second time around. I found a strappy pale green chiffon cocktail dress for under $200 with a matching wrap necessary for the church ceremony. I got it on a quick trip to the mall. I was self-assured enough to know what I wanted this time around—enough to make a quick decision. I still enjoy wearing the dress—it's elegant and sexy."

Francesca, fifty-two, Edina, Minnesota

"I'm getting married in three weeks and still don't have the dress. At first, I wanted to wear an elegant pantsuit because I'm a pants type of girl, but my mom insisted I wear a dress. My fiancé wants me to wear a dress, too. So *voilà*, a dress it is! Even though I haven't been married before, I'll be wearing color against my mother's orders. I have a more utilitarian perspective when it comes to my wardrobe, so I want to wear something that I love and can wear again and again."

Elaine, forty-four, interior designer and author, Manhattan

"When I remarried at the age of forty-four, I opted not to wear white. I decided on a knee-length cocktail dress in a burnt orange color, which looked especially beautiful when we married at sunset on a beach in Hawaii. I say go for color that you feel fabulous and sexy in!"

Marilyn, sales and jewelry design, Livermore, California

"I got married when I was forty-seven. I wore a white pantsuit that I already had in my closet. It just seemed right for the occasion and happened to fit. Someone mistakenly burned a hole in its lapel while smoking that day. I'm so glad I didn't buy something new."

Lise, fifty-four, attorney, Providence, Rhode Island

I often think of a college friend's aplomb when she wore scarlet petticoats under white. She clearly enjoyed who she was and was confident enough not to wear what her mother thought was proper. She got it right: She is still embracing herself and the man she first married decades ago.

I haven't a clue what I would wear. Would I be practical and attempt to find something already in my closet? Would I wear separates like I did the first time around? Likely it will be something entirely unexpected, as most fresh starts are.

Closet Confidential: Dressing From the Inside Out

"The first time I married for reasons from the outside in, which was a disaster. The second time I got it right—I fell in love from the inside out. My second husband and I had been together fourteen years before we started a discussion about getting married.

"Early one June morning we decided to stop by the courthouse and get information about what documents would be required to get a marriage certificate. We had many other errands to take care of that day so we were the first ones at the recorder's office.

"The woman we spoke with told us what was required and said she had time right then to marry us. Would we be interested? We said, sure, why not. We entered her office and stood in front of her, holding hands while she read generic vows to us. Behind her was a large map of the County of Marin from the early 1950s. We could hear cars driving in and out of the parking lot right below her window.

"As she continued to read, however, the world around us seemed to change. I felt filled with light and peace. The plain office and the asphalt parking lot seemed to get very large and luminescent. Our hearts were filled with love and the room radiated warmth and authentic spirituality. As I gazed into my husband's eyes I realized that this was the perfect wedding."

Susan, sixty, artist, Point Reyes Station, California

25

Mother of the Bride or Groom

Our goal is to look our very best for this life-defining moment. After all, the ceremony concedes that our children are moving on with their lives. So are we. These milestones also hold a mirror to who we are now as women. As our daughters tap into their inner woman, we connect to our inner girl. We want to feel pretty, feminine, elegant, beautiful, and appropriate.

> ### Closet Confidential: Dress for You
>
> "I lost weight for my son's wedding. I wore a long copper-colored flamingo-styled dress that was tight and had ruffles that started from mid-hip. It had three-quarter sleeves and was low-cut, but I had it modified to not show too much cleavage and to reveal more of my shoulders. Shoulders are so sexy. I wore earth tones for my makeup with smoky eyes and hair extensions so my hair was long which I think is youthful. I wore long earrings with lots of stones, and gold platform shoes for comfort. I had been planning on wearing a bright color for the dress because it was in summer and I was tanned, but I realized that I am the mother and should wear a more serious color. But I also wanted to say that I am a sexy mother (of four) and grandmother and that 'life continues and I'm still here,' but not in a distasteful way."
>
> **Doris, forty-nine, construction company owner, Queens, New York**

> "My son's wedding was formal and I thought it was going to be tedious finding a dress. I started at Bergdorf and there it was. A long straight column of white and blue (my favorite color) with spaghetti straps and ruffles in front. I had shoes dyed to match and wore a pashmina to cover my shoulders. I didn't consult with the mother of the bride—she's ten years younger and beautiful. I couldn't compete so I did my own thing. I wasn't going to wear beige and keep my mouth shut. I love the dress and have worn it several times since."
>
> *Betsy, fifty-nine, New Canaan, Connecticut*

Dressing to compete with the bride, upstage the bride, or in an overtly sexy or seductive manner is vulgar. When we think of sex at a wedding, it should be about the virgin bride and her wedding night, not the wayward mom.

But dowdy is old, and we are not old, and we are not invisible. The mother of the bride today often appears young and fit. We can show some skin—a bit of cleavage, some back, a strapless neckline, great legs—rather than cover ourselves up in a confection of pastels. Some religious ceremonies require covering the arms. A pretty wrap will do the job.

W2W Closet Journal: Our Children's Weddings

When imagining what to wear for any special occasion, write down how you want to *feel* and what you want your clothes to communicate.

_____

_____

_____

_____

_____

W2W Closet Practice: The Plan

Planning what to wear as mother of the bride or groom is much like planning for our own wedding. Consider it an opportunity to get out of a closet and beauty rut and take a fresh look at how you've been pulling yourself together.

Many mothers of the bride or groom stay clear of the bridal department and choose to have a dress made. They want a hand in creating how they appear. For others, their priority is to find a dress or dressy suit they can enjoy wearing for other occasions in the future. For the maximum options in the least amount of time, make an appointment with personal shoppers at several different stores (a complimentary service in many stores and boutiques). Let them know in advance roughly what you are looking for—long, short, pants, dress, suit—depending on the venue and your personal comfort.

Choose to wear a color that is flattering, rather than coordinate with the wedding party. Indeed, it is not uncommon today for mothers of the bride or groom to wear black for timeless chic.

Closet Confidential: Shop Prepared

"It's hard to have fun shopping for a dress for any special occasion, especially as the mother of the bride or groom when you need to keep color schemes and other rules in mind. If you shop wearing short socks, a baggy bra and underpants, bad hair, and no makeup, you are setting yourself up to feel bad before you start.

"Please, do yourself the favor of wearing your Spanx or control-top pantyhose and a great bra, preferably strapless. And wear some makeup! You know the feeling when you're at the hairdresser with your head wrapped in a towel, you have no makeup on, and you have to stare at yourself in the mirror. You don't need to feel that way in the dressing room."

Kay Unger, fashion designer

Many mothers diet and up their exercise. Some even undergo cosmetic surgery—just don't do it within a year of the event in case of long-term swelling or other possible side effects.

Heads up! Never make major changes to your hair just before a special occasion. "I recommend to women before they make a drastic change to come in for styling. Blow-drying your hair in different ways—straight, wavy, curly—can look and feel like a new haircut," says Edita Evon of the Warren-Tricomi Salon in Greenwich, Connecticut. If you plan on experimenting with your hair, give it plenty of time for adjustments. A year is ideal.

Also visit makeup counters for complimentary makeovers. When you find a look you like and a makeup artist you trust, make an appointment with her to do your makeup the day of the wedding—or better still, to teach you how to apply it yourself. Show her what you are going to wear in advance, as it may impact the choice of makeup colors.

It's also a good idea to have a dress rehearsal (keep price tags on). Have yourself photographed so you can critique the overall look with an analytical eye. After all, wedding pictures have a long life.

26

But You Don't Look
Like a Grandmother

My mother's best friend would constantly tell anyone who would listen, "The worst thing about being a grandmother is sleeping with a grandfather." I considered it Borscht Belt humor even though she wasn't Jewish and lived in Europe, but perhaps it's not surprising that her husband had a mistress—chicken or egg?

My mother didn't want to be called grandma, so she came up with an acronym—GG (Grandma Gerd, her birth name). My daughters misunderstood, thinking she didn't want to be a grandmother. My mother loves and enjoys her six grandchildren but isn't defined by them. Nor does she want to "look" like a grandmother.

But what does a grandmother look like today?

Women no longer allow themselves to be narrowly defined by any role, but are enriched by and dress for each of them.

> ### *Closet Confidential: Dressing for Life*
> Aline expanded her workout wardrobe when she took up yoga and weight lifting to be stronger, have better balance, and enjoy more confidence when carrying her grandchild up and down stairs.
>
> *Aline, seventy-nine, Pittsburgh*

"I will not wear what my grandmother used to wear just because I am a grammy! I keep my appearance in perspective. I know I am not twenty-five or thirty anymore, however, I refuse to wear clothes that cover me from head to toe! I constantly work on keeping weight off. I deserve to show off my body a little."

Brenda, fifty, executive assistant, Frisco, Texas

"I don't fit into the stereotypical image of what my Grandmother looked like. In some ways it is a very liberating age. I can do things for myself that I didn't have the time or know-how twenty years ago. I now dress casually and comfortably. I am always looking for jeans with stretch that fit well."

Donna, forty-nine, charity organizer, Dallas

My mother was eighty-one when she was inspired to buy her first pair of jeans and Pumas after trekking Machu Picchu.

You may be a grandmother, but you are also a woman. Dress for your life. When you're playing with your grandchildren, wear comfortable clothes that you can later throw in the wash, and shoes you can run around in. When you are dressing for a night out, kick it up a notch or two.

There is never a reason to dress boringly whatever your age. Style rules don't expire with age: Wear flattering clothes that fit well, are comfortable, and that you enjoy wearing. Have fun with color and accessories. Try on new styles of clothes and different colors when you shop. If something makes you feel like a grannie or too young, stay away from it. It's important to feel good in your clothes, but even more important to feel good in your skin.

Personally, I can't wait to be a grandmother. Like becoming a mother of the bride or groom, it is an affirmation that life continues. For our children it's filled with the excitement of possibilities. For us it's more about bearing witness to the joy of now. It gives us pause to reflect on our own lives, the passage of time we have experienced, and our contribution to this celebration of the future.

27

Relax, It's Only a Mini-Pause

*For everything its season and for every activity under
heaven its time:
a time to embrace and a time to refrain from embracing,
a time to seek and a time to lose,
a time to keep and a time to cast away,
a time to rend and a time to mend . . .*

Ecclesiastes 3:1–7

The Joy of Closet

In a 2005 study, Penn State researchers analyzed the responses of women between thirty-five and fifty-five in a survey on body image and concluded that the emphasis on being young and thin in our culture has more impact on our sexual functioning and satisfaction than menopause. Who knew that a Feel-Good Closet could also contribute to your orgasm?

What we wear can help us feel pretty or sensual or attractive and confident, but only if we are in sync with our body, whatever its size.

Closet Confidential: *Body-Confidence*

"Dressing sexy in a size 14 is an oxymoron. I can tell you that at my weight, I don't feel good in anything or nothing. I know it is a state of mind, but I am so upset with myself that I don't feel comfortable in any of my clothes. I don't know whether to go to AA or Weight Watchers!"

Lise, fifty-four, attorney, Providence, Rhode Island

> "My husband always tells me I look beautiful and never criticizes my weight. When I caught him having a serious affair, I thanked God that I had been taking care of myself. I think I would have killed myself otherwise."
>
> *Ali, thirty-nine, Feng Shui consultant, Brooklyn, New York*

> "A lot of women use turning sixty as an excuse to give up on themselves. But for others of us, it's why we work on what we work on. I do Iyengar yoga two or three times a week. It's important for strength and balance as we age."
>
> *Betsy, sixty-four, Ketchum, Idaho*

If my fat cells were distributed more abundantly in my breasts than my stomach, I think I would be hot, and not just in flashes. As our bodies evolve in their own unique way, none of us can escape the natural life cycle of menopause. It's hard to feel great when we are besieged by hormonal changes that can cause fatigue, sleepless nights, memory loss, apathy, weight gain, the resettling of body mass, lagging libido, vaginal dryness, and a roller coaster of emotions.

And it wreaks havoc on our closet. Even if we still fit into our clothes, many of them no longer feel comfortable. My knit sweaters that were once cozy now feel feverous to wear. And forget turtlenecks—if it's a choice between having a fiery face and covering my neck, comfort trumps camouflage.

Closet Confidential: *Crossing the Great Divide*

> "Menopause is reshaping my body. I am using yoga twice a week to keep a more svelte figure. I have pared down the volume and weight of clothes, and have found that stretch fabrics, especially in pants, look great. I am also wearing clothes with clean lines and in softer solid colors, which look much better than prints."
>
> *Sandra*

"Four years after breast cancer put me into menopause, I continue to dress in layers. I gave away my heavy winter coats, and my wool slacks and sweaters. When I shop for clothes, it's a question of will they manage my hot flashes. Can I take a top layer off quickly without ruining my makeup? Can I launder rather than dry clean? My wardrobe hardly changes with the seasons since I am always hot. It mostly consists of sweater sets in cotton, silk, or those in a combination of lightweight fabrics. I just vary the colors and try to stay cool! I've even started a sleepwear company using fabrics that wick moisture away from the body, so I can feel dry and comfortable when I sleep at night."

Haralee, fifty-three, Portland, Oregon

"I was falling apart in menopause, but I didn't realize it at the time. I had other very stressful mid-life crises to deal with—divorce, finances, professional turmoil. When I gained weight I thought it must be restaurant food because that was the kind of life I was living then. I even broke my metatarsal without noticing until I couldn't wear a shoe. But I did notice that a lot of my friends also looked like they fell apart in their fifties, but then they, and me, got through it in about five years."

Kathryn, sixty-five, writer, Manhattan

"When menopause hit, so did the extra pounds. I started wearing big loose-fitting tops to hide my lack of figure until I decided to wear shorter tops that were slightly more fitted. I not only looked better, I felt better about myself. That's when the pounds started coming off."

Collie, fifty-seven, sales, Cedar Lake, Michigan

Lost and Found

Style is about surviving having been through a lot and making it look easy. —C. Z. Guest

It's more than our closets that transition into menopause. There are many major life shifts that catapult us into uncharted waters—a change in family dynamics, career status, health, economics, or relationships. Many of us feel like we are no longer the women we were. We aren't. Life intrudes upon the old habits and closets that had defined us for decades.

The metamorphosis can be turbulent, as it was in puberty, but like then it compels us to regroup and redefine the next part of our lives. We rewrote the cultural norms as we grew into women, just as we are creating the new cultural landscape of our lives today. Many of us emerge like a Phoenix, feeling energized—stronger, wiser, sexier, more confident—and back in sync with our closet.

Closet Confidential: *Breaking Closet Habits*

"I loosened up in what I wore after I lost my baby. It wasn't fair that I gained baby weight and lactated, but didn't have my baby. I wanted to start fresh. I was slow to wear prints and now I wear them with a vengeance."

Beatriz, forty-nine, CEO of HispanAmérica and power yoga teacher, Newfoundland, Pennsylvania

"After I was diagnosed with the early stages of melanoma, I changed the way I dress. My first response was to swathe myself in fabric, which made me look more like a beekeeper than an elegant professional. My workplace is casual, but I began to delight in dressing up. Great tailoring, fine fabrics, and jewelry are my fashion epiphany. Hats have become my signature. I dress to express my individuality, style, and confidence."

Sunny, nonprofit executive, Los Angeles

"I lost twenty-five pounds on the South Beach Diet. My new body was my sixtieth-birthday gift to myself. Before I had this feeling in the back of my mind that I had lost something. When I lost the weight, I realized what I had lost and found. I remembered what it was like to feel good in my body. Now I feel like I can wear anything, but my daughters caution me against dressing inappropriately young."

Marilyn, sixty-plus, Internet entrepreneur, Chatham, New York

"I've gotten more casual since my husband died. When you don't live with anyone you can wear what you like, even the same thing every day. Recently, an acquaintance remarked that my handwriting looked artistic, and asked if I paint or draw. I told her I used to, but hadn't pursued either since my husband had been renowned for these talents. She responded, 'Well, you don't have that excuse anymore.' I thought her comment a bit harsh, but of course she was right. She provoked me to fool around with photography again, something I had enjoyed a long time ago. I've also had a book published for the first time. It's a paradox that the profound sadness of my husband's death sparked my creativity."

Diane, sixty-four, design writer, Manhattan

"My life is a new adventure for my husband and me. The passion is back. We have moved to a ranch after living our lives in cities. I now spend a lot of time in my garden, which is a good place to strip back to the essentials. I am in touch with nature—the deer knocking down the fence that holds the cattle, the aggravating bird that is nesting on the house, dealing with the coyotes and our dogs, and living by the seasons—it's all great. These are things I had never considered. Before menopause, we are naturally in touch with our cycles. Now, after menopause, living so close to nature has gotten me in touch with its cycles, which to me are a life force. There is now a harmony in all aspects of my life."

Julia, fifty-plus, art consultant, Richfield, Idaho

W2W Closet Practice: Fresh Starts

Now is the time to reimagine and reclaim your closet—to Assess, Dejunk, and Renew. You can't make room for the new if you're hanging on to the old. But what's old? It's not necessarily the years some things have been in your closet, but whether they fit your new life, and sense of self.

Fresh Start 1. Clean Your Closet

After leaving my job as a governor's legal counsel, I went home to clean out my closet. I had been looking forward to doing that for twenty years.

—Claire, Providence, Rhode Island

Fresh Start 2. Closet Therapy

When I feel bummed, I clean out my closet while watching a favorite movie over and over again. It's a restorative lull. I am aware that there's something brewing in my subconscious and it will be followed by a huge surge of creativity. It's a way of regrouping, while being conscious that I'm figuring out what's next.

> —Susan, fifty-something, mother of four and former Manhattan advertising executive, West Marin, California

Fresh Start 3. Prioritize

I am between jobs. There are ranges of possibilities that are presenting themselves to me. I am excited, but experience fear and trepidation. If I don't work, then I won't be able to buy Chanel suits on sale anymore. But I am enjoying this hiatus. It's the first time in a very long while that I am taking care of me. It was always about my children and work, and now they're grown. I had neglected my dating life all these years. I don't need to marry, but now I am ready for a relationship with a man.

> —Andrea, fifty-plus, business executive, Manhattan

Fresh Start 4. Get Engaged

Hitting fifty wasn't so bad until I had an age-related injury and was forced to close my dance business. That's when I first felt mortal. In the subsequent three years, I gained eight pounds eating sweets and drinking alcohol while I convalesced. That all changed when I found something I enjoyed doing. My husband bought a company and wanted me to design the office space. I became totally engaged. Having a project made time intense again. I felt useful which made me feel satisfied. To design a successful office space, I needed to listen to the needs of those who worked there. I felt like I was giving back to the world again.

Now I express myself with clothes and enjoy playing dress-up, something I had never done before. At first I started by wearing frilly skirts, but now I'm back to wearing black and white, so I can dress them up with accessories. I have an addiction for funky earrings, and I shop all over the world for handmade, expressive jewelry.

—Sheelah, fifty-seven, interior designer, Rye, New York

Fresh Start 5. Adapt

My style hasn't evolved. It's always been tailored, but the colors changed depending on where I lived. I grew up in Rye, New York, wearing preppy clothes, which were colorful. Then after several years of being married with children in Virginia, we moved to Connecticut. I love color, but wore more black clothes there because I lived closer to New York City. Now that our kids are on their own, we've moved out west so my husband could pursue his next career as an avid fisherman. I feel comfortable wearing the same style of clothes here that I would wear in New Canaan, New York City, or San Francisco, where my grandchildren live. When they're simple in solid colors, they are easier to dress up with different kinds of jewelry.

—Betsy, sixty-four, Ketchum, Idaho

Fresh Start 6. Reimagine

When I turn sixty-five, I am going to reinvent myself. I want to retire to a great new life—a new chapter as an older woman. It's easy to get stuck in the way you care for yourself. You have to physically break the pattern for change. I want a big change. I am going to cut my hair short and dye it platinum. I am going to start ballroom dancing again, an activity I had enjoyed, but stopped when I was fifty. I wasn't inspired to move my feet at the time.

—Goldie, sixty-plus, health care administrative assistant, Yonkers, New York

Fresh Start 7. Tidy Up

My husband and I now live in the country and work at home. We often go for days seeing no one but each other; nonetheless, I dress. Not dress up. But dress well. Good jeans or corduroys and attractive sweaters and scarves—the French woman's secret weapon—in good colors (not always dark; the weather here is gloomy enough; besides, the older I get, the better pale colors look on me). We both make an effort.

—Marilyn, sixty-plus, Internet entrepreneur, Chatham, New York

Fresh Start 8. Have Fun

I had personal uniforms when I was working and had to get lots of things done in a short amount of time, including getting dressed. In the 1980s I wore corporate suits. For my last job it was Levi's 501s with decorative tops. Now that I'm on less of a schedule, I ask myself in the morning: What do I feel like wearing? What is my mood? I'm much more into fun clothes now. I've gotten into wearing comfortable pants in colorful wacky patterns that are easy to pull on. I wear them with simple tops that are flattering, and amusing earrings. It's my thing; it's become what people expect to see me in.

—Susan, fifty-something, mother of four and former Manhattan advertising executive, West Marin, California

Fresh Start 9. Find a Balance

I don't want to wear only a pencil skirt and high heels and I never want to wear a navy suit again, but I want to live a life that is more than just jeans.

—Terry, forty-six, financial consultant, Manhattan

Fresh Start 10. Brave New You

Funny, as I've gotten older, I feel less compelled to follow norms. I am questioning conformity and convention at every turn. I want to speak more freely, dress less and less conventionally, and my haircuts get more interesting every month. In terms of my career, I keep finding new ones. I love being a full-time business owner and marketing strategist, but I also love teaching yoga now, too.

—Beatriz, forty-nine, CEO of HispanAmérica and power yoga teacher, Pennsylvania

Fresh Start 11.
Never Give Up on You or Your Closet!

I see how some women just give up and accept the body they have, and there is a certain amount of peace in that. Others, like me, have gone from size 6 to 12 and don't want to get to size 16, so we work out. But it's important for all of us to dress to play up our assets while camouflaging our stomach, our thighs, our hips, whatever is growing out of control.

—Lynne, sixty, retail consultant, Charleston, West Virginia

Fresh Start 12.
Dress for Today and for the Rest of Your Life

When I was diagnosed with breast cancer, I dressed to look great each time I went to the oncologist. I wanted the doctor to get the message that I was going to live.

—Susan, fifty-something, mother of four, West Marin, California

28

A Closet for the Rest of Your Life

Look in the mirror less, and feel more. —Bobbi Brown

This book began with my bikini crisis and closet betrayal, the close of my business, my divorce, and the terror that I was entering an unimaginable new time in my life. The trajectory of my life had been derailed. I felt like I was falling down a rabbit hole, much like Alice in Wonderland, unprepared for what was next.

I have since traveled through perimenopause into menopause, with additional weight gain, the onset of the Alien, credit card debt, and a futile attempt to self-medicate—wine and martinis were the placebos of choice.

I thought in the aftermath of divorce, the family dramas would be over, but the recovery was brutal for all of us. I was no longer declarative about much of anything—except in my core, I knew a bad pattern had to be broken before we could all heal and move on. But the beliefs I had long held and the everyday realities that I had come to count on had crumbled. It's no wonder I lost touch with my closet—I lost touch with me!

Keep going. No matter what happens in life, just keep going.
—Tina Turner, sixty-five

My grandmother taught me to pray when I was a young girl. My prayers had always been of thanksgiving, especially in dark times. Over this recent rough period, I was praying a lot.

My loved ones rallied.

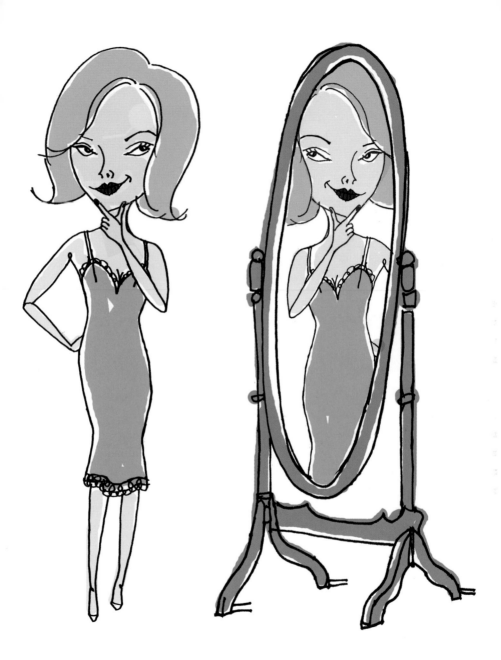

Friends called me daily, while others were simply there, whether I needed to talk or be silent. They welcomed me into their homes for holidays I couldn't share with my daughters, because of visitation rights.

They invited me into their book clubs, which got me out of my solitude and into the company of other women. After lively book discussions, there was girl talk. When I shared my closet crises, they shared theirs. The closet became a metaphor for everything else going on in our lives. By sharing our experiences and collective wisdom—as we were physically and psychically adjusting to a new time in our lives—we were letting one another know: It's okay, we're in this together and we'll get through it together!

Colleagues got me focused professionally. They designed and printed transitional business cards for me, coaxed me to write my "mission statement," and pushed me into the door of *More Magazine* to write a column that would sharpen my voice for this book. They encouraged me to share my journey and those of other women to inspire and empower us all to move into this next part of our lives gracefully and confidently.

My mother considers traveling the next best thing to buying a dress when spirits need a boost, so we traveled together. But it is her strength of spirit that really inspired me to get out of my funk. When my father died and her investments were swindled, she was the age I am now. She had to find her own voice to survive. She grew young, strong, and independent. She found a new career in real estate, became a devoted trustee at Old Westbury Gardens, and became a glamorous do-it-yourself hostess and a globe-trotting adventurer—all on a tight budget—and an upbeat enthusiast to generations of friends. She also fell in love again.

The bonds between my sisters and me strengthened. Jill and her boyfriend at the time included me in their world of fun friends and weekend getaways. Their lifeline roped me out of bed. Susan and her husband, Philip, gave me safe harbor for long stretches of time in their home on the other side of the country. Spending time with my nieces and nephew helped to rejuvenate my spirit.

I developed a visceral connection to the raw natural beauty of the land where they live. I relished the dramatic changes of weather in natural canyons, rather than just tolerating it in the cement-and-glass canyons I was accustomed to. The fear of no longer needing a morning alarm clock gave way to loving the freedom of being released from its assault. Living closer to the natural rhythms of nature nourished me.

I wore feel-good clothes to hike, write, cook, and sleep in. They were simple, cozy, and practical—a balance of aesthetics and function, much like a No. 2 pencil. I adorned them with the big gold hoop earrings, over-size wooden ring, and crystal heart necklace that had become my closet favorites wherever I was.

When I told a fashionista friend that "fashion" and the fashion police weren't meaningful to me anymore, she was astonished. I tried to explain that I still enjoy feeling happy in what I wear, but what that meant was changing. I had spent a lifetime espousing the idea that if you looked good, you would feel good. Now feeling good for me helped me look great, at least when I faced my mirror and my closet. What else really counts?

During this time of gestation, a friend recommended a psychiatrist for me to see. No, not because of my changing views on "fashion," but to help me sort out the mini-tsunami of life changes I was coping with. Finding the right shrink is much like finding a personal shopper or going on a blind date. It can be a non-plus or a horror, but when it clicks, it's a gift.

This doctor was not reticent. She was relentless in forcing me to emerge from a haze of confusion by digging deep within myself to find my voice and articulate it. It was a series of (expensive) baby steps, but each session felt monumental. I was finding my way.

Another friend gave me a few books on Buddhism. I am not a Buddhist, but I found comfort in some of the teachings. A basic tenet is that suffering ceases when desire ceases. That's only possible when you abandon ego and live fully in the now, not in the want of the future or the longing for the past.

Buddha was a storyteller. A particular story that I heard during this time resonated: A monk set off on a long pilgrimage to find the Buddha. He devoted many years to his search until he finally reached the land where the Buddha was said to live. While crossing the river to this country, the monk looked around as the boatman rowed.

He noticed something floating toward them. As it got closer, he realized that it was the corpse of a person. When it drifted so close that he could almost touch it, he suddenly recognized the dead body.

It was his own! He lost all control and wailed at the sight of himself, still and lifeless, drifting along the river's currents. That moment was the beginning of his liberation.

I was also galvanized by a passage in Suzanne Braun Levine's book *Inventing the Rest of Our Lives: Women in Second Adulthood:*

When we gather for fiftieth and sixtieth birthdays, we ask each other if we are grown up yet. The answer is: Yes, we are grown up, but at the same time we are only halfway there. We are about to grow up again.

Reading this was an Oprah "aha!" moment for me. Wow! Was I a babe—okay, baby—on this leg of the journey?

In the movie *What the Bleep Do We Know!?*, there was a scene where the character played by actress Marlee Matlin was filled with self-loathing because she perceived the woman she saw in the mirror as fat. The next scene portrayed a shift in her perspective: She adorned her body with love notes—a way of "dressing" to honor it in the present.

Hmmmm. I could look into the mirror with old eyes, or with new eyes. (No, not an eye-lift.) Instead of mourning what was, I began to open up to new possibilities. I started to get excited about the "adventure" I was in—the adventure of my life.

I Dejunked the Burden of Ego

I am no longer a 118-pound cover girl (scary in retrospect), but I got over that decades ago.

I am no longer the 135-pound tall blond wife of childbearing age (well, I am still tall, and blond with help).

I am no longer a career fashionista whose closet is packed with the latest in fashion and credit card debt to match.

I am no longer living outside my means, but within them, and have found happiness in that. I have fun again in what I wear and feel less stress.

I am no longer a perimenopausal daughter wearing two-piece bathing suits, but I am stronger and more fit today than I've been at most other times in my life, even if I am also heavier.

I am no longer in dread of falling to the bottom of the rabbit hole, because I landed and picked myself up and have received so many blessings along the way.

Since the Alien found its way into my closet, it has talked to me every day. And I have responded. I exercise for it. I dress for it. I am humbled by it. I no longer regard it as an Alien, but as my Buddha belly, a reminder (thank you, Dad) to honor my body, whatever its size, shape, age, or health, and to enjoy dressing it up!

I have since taken surfing, windsurfing, and rowing lessons. I defied all expectations by successfully rolling a kayak in white water. I've rekindled my love of playing tennis even though I have lost my game. I walk, hike, and bike, and in the winter cross-country ski and snowshoe everywhere whenever possible.

I've started swimming again and I've learned to bike with clip-on shoes (initially way scary) and to train for my first triathlon, which I completed (without losing a pound)!

Practicing hot yoga remains the best way for me to nurture myself. It gives me strength and flexibility, cleanses my body and mind, and requires being present, at one, with my body without judgment, but with loving-kindness. It's an added blessing for me when I practice with my daughter Carolyn, who is an avid enthusiast. Any shared experience with either of my two girls is worth gold to me.

I still get mistaken in exercise class for being pregnant. Nonetheless I am having fun with my body, even when it's bruised, bandaged, iced up, aching, or appears not as fit as I feel. And I feel as though I've tapped into my inner girl, the one filled the wonder and enthusiasm, but she's smarter with the wisdom of the woman I have grown into.

And I am loving the changes in my closet. As I was rebuilding my life, I was reconfiguring my closet.

The way I see it, if you want the rainbow, you gotta put up with the rain. —Dolly Parton

So, What Am I Going to Wear for the Rest of My Life?

The "labels" in my closet have tipped from Armani to REI. Sleek active sportswear and athletic shoes are as important to me now as designer suits and pumps were during my career in fashion. The mix of what my Feel-Good Closet holds now is expressive of the mix of my life. When I hike, I still want to dress like a woman—fun earrings and splashes of pretty colors do the job.

I make sure nowadays to wear everything in my Feel-Good Closet. The Hermès silk scarf that I hijacked from my mother's closet as a young fashion editor now makes for a very chic bandanna when I'm cross-country skiing—did you know that silk keeps you very warm?

If something has been unworn for a while, I move it front and center in my closet and make a supreme effort to wear it with the clothes I keep reaching for. It's another way of shopping my closet. If I'm still not wearing it, I recycle it, so someone else might enjoy it.

Rather than be the curator of my closet, I have made it my partner. I enjoy getting dressed again, even if there are times that minding my closet feels like I'm repairing a roof—spending money on orthotics, reading glasses, the latest in body-shaping underwear, and who knows what next. But my closet helps me to feel:

Flirtatious. I've never been a flirt, but I now want flirtation in my closet. It's fun feeling girlie! Much to my daughters' horror, I often wear skirts and dresses with patterned hosiery and high boots or kicky shoes. And I'm always looking for tops that show off my shoulders or those with some sort of decorative embellishment to cover up my middle.

Happy. My closet and I are having more fun together—it's the inner diva in me. Adding one unexpected item to the mix—an oversize piece of faux jewelry, anything in an animal print, a splash of energizing color, a decorative scarf, an amusing accessory—makes us both smile.

Adventurous. Techno fabrics with varying amounts of stretch and sheen is a valiant attempt to sculpt my body in styles worthy of an *Avengers* remake. Wearing electric colors, strategically placed, energizes me even before I step foot on a hiking trail.

Besides the great look, the supreme comfort, and the fantasies active wear inspires, basic wardrobe rules apply—form follows function. The goal is to wear what helps my body function at its peak performance—keep it dry, cool or warm, vented and padded for protection. **Comfortable.** White jeans, skirts, black pants and tops made in feel-good fabrics—denim with stretch, cashmere, Polarfleece, cotton—are the basics I keep reaching for even though the fit and styles will continue to change.

I like the simplicity of my closet and that it's geared for all sorts of adventures, but I am careful not to be complacent again in my relationship with me, my closet, or anyone else. If my closet feels stuck in a rut, it means that I am. That is not a signal to run out and buy new clothes, but I should take a fresh look at what I am wearing and why. It's important to be absorbed, not self-absorbed, in a world bigger than a closet.

Inner Style

I have recently been spending more time out west, in a part of the country where when you're asked what you do, it's not about your profession, but if you prefer to fly-fish, hike, backpack, ski backcountry, downhill, or cross-country, road bike, mountain bike, skeet shoot, hunt, kayak, and/or canoe.

I was dining in a restaurant in this western town when I noticed a glass on the bar that held several reading glasses for patrons like me who cannot negotiate a menu without wearing a pair. It made me laugh at how there were so many of us living this next part our lives, which is a delicate balance between the adventure and the reality that will continue to impact on our closets as our bodies and lives unfold in ways none of us can know. The walking stick I use today when I hike mountains might very well help me navigate around my home tomorrow—presumably a more stylish version.

In nature, nothing is perfect and everything is perfect. Trees can be contorted, bent in weird ways, and they're still beautiful. —Alice Walker

A Feel-Good Closet can't guarantee romance, a successful career, weight loss, excellent health, a fountain of youth, or that you can wear stilettos comfortably again. And I wish I could tell you that finding my Feel-Good Closet means I've lost weight, am off all medication, am completely out of debt, and have found black pants and white jeans that fit perfectly!

But as I have gotten back in sync with my closet, I've gotten back in sync with me. My asthma medication has been halved, as has my debt; my cholesterol is lower; and I am training for my next triathlon.

I have finally learned that nothing in life is perfect. Good enough is great! If we are obsessive about our closets, we will never be pleased. If we are neglectful, we are punishing ourselves. But when we are mindful, we can be content.

I like the way I feel in my clothes again. I enjoy the fashionista in me (I guess she will always be there in some capacity), but there comes a time to stop talking about clothes and live a life in them. My closet thrives with life now rather than striving for a life.

And that's part of its beauty. By being engaged in life and the messiness of it all (and dressing for it!), we continue to grow rather than grow old. Like Alice, I've come to appreciate that there will always be something new to marvel at and dress for in the rabbit hole. And I suspect that I'll always be in search of black pants and white jeans that fit!

By the way, as my body continues to evolve, I no longer feel great wearing the bikini, but I try not to beat myself up about it, either. I liken it to a toxic relationship. Sometimes you just need to know when to let go.

Style-wise, most of us eventually look better in a one-piece swimsuit, and the reality is that I've never felt great wearing a two-piece. But I've come to realize that the bathing suit that so appalled my mother got me back into my closet to Assess, Dejunk, and Renew its contents, which forced me on this journey to take a fresh look at my life. Those two simple pieces of fabric helped me to let go of the promise of youth, and learn to honor and enjoy the body I live in today.

So I wear my bathing suit today (now a black suck-me-in one-piece) like Aunt Katje, with big hoop earrings, kicky sandals, and a sarong. And my mother is at ease that I share my closet with someone who loves me—Buddha Belly and all—and tells me, "You're beautiful, and you look great, too!"

There is no end. There is no beginning. There is only the passion of life. —Federico Fellini

I find it difficult to end this book. As my daughter Carolyn counseled, "There is no ending, Mom." She's right. Writing this book has been a *charrette*—there will always be more women to talk with, more stories to share, more to refine, delete, mend, tailor, much like our closets, and our lives.

Our closets hold our DNA—they tell our story. They are a link between generations. A friend's young daughter-in-law remarked after we recently met, "Kim's so interesting and chic." My closet and my Buddha belly rejoice in that. And it made me smile, because that's how many people describe my mother. My mother's closet, and those of other women, continue to inspire my journey, however different the paths we dress for may be. My daughters occasionally borrow from mine as they create their own closets and find their own Style and Life Mentors. And my memory closet grows, however ruthlessly I dejunk. As with any good friend, it's memories that bind us together, tangible or not.

How about you?

Go back into your closet and continue the conversation as you dress for the rest of your life.

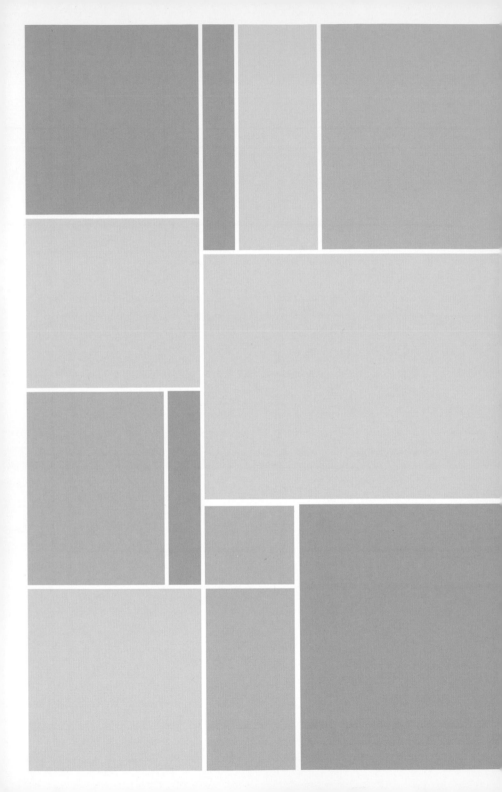

There came a
time when the
risk to remain
tight in the bud
was more painful
than the risk it
took to blossom.

—Anaïs Nin

WARDROBE WISDOM

The trick is in what
one emphasizes.
We either make
ourselves
miserable, or we
make ourselves
happy. The
amount of work is
the same.

—Carlos Castaneda

Recommended Reading

Audrey Style and *Jackie Style*, by Pamela Clarke Keogh (HarperCollins, 1999, 2001) are as entertaining, glamorous, and insightful as their subjects.

Bobbi Brown Living Beauty, by Bobbi Brown (Springboard Press, 2007). Written in celebration of her fiftieth birthday. Brown shares beauty advice for our changing skin and encourages us to honor our laugh lines and age gracefully.

Comfort Me with Apples: More Adventures at the Table (Random House, 2002), and other books by Ruth Reichl, share her ravenous appetite for a delicious life.

Does This Make Me Look Fat? by Leah Feldon (Villard, 2000). Leah goes past the questions to the answers.

Eat, Pray, Love, by Elizabeth Gilbert (Penguin, 2006). How can you argue with the three best things in life?

Fifty on Fifty, by Bonnie Miller Rubin (Warner, 1998). Allegedly inspired when Bonnie looked into the mirror of a dressing room while trying on a bathing suit—what is it about bathing suits?

The 5 Principles of Ageless Living, by supermodel Dayle Haddon (Atria, 2003) is a physical and spiritual energy boost.

Going Gray: What I Learned About Beauty, Sex, Work, Motherhood, Authenticity, and Everything Else That Really Matters, by Anne Kreamer (Little, Brown, 2007). Deciding to gray or not to gray? This is a "real" friend to help you sort out the difference between gray and silver.

The Good Body, by Eve Ensler (Villard, 2005). With wit, candor, and unflinching honesty, Ensler gives perspective to how women view their changing bodies.

Inventing the Rest of Our Lives: Women in Second Adulthood, by Suzanne Braun Levine (Viking, 2005), was my "aha!" moment.

The Places That Scare You: A Guide to Fearlessness in Difficult Times (and audiotapes) (Shambala, 2001), by Pema Chodron, opened my heart and my eyes.

The Red Hat Society: Fun and Friendship After Fifty, by Sue Ellen Cooper and Andrea Reekstin (Warner Books, 2004). Feel like you're alone or disappearing? Check this out.

A Round-Heeled Woman: My Late-Life Adventures in Sex and Romance, by Jane Juska (Villard, 2004). The author published a classified ad that read: "Before I turn sixty-seven—next March—I would like to have a lot of sex with a man I like. If you want to talk first, Trollope works for me." A romping read.

Secrets of a Fashion Therapist: What You Can Learn Behind the Dressing Room Door, by Betty Halbreich (Collins Living, 2005). The legendary personal shopper at Bergdorf Goodman wittily shares style advice.

The Silent Passage: Menopause, by Gail Sheehy (Pocket, revised edition, 1998). I was reading this while waiting in a bar for a friend, when a man started to chat me up, thinking the book would be a conversation starter—menopause isn't flirtatious, but it can be amusing.

Why I Wore Lipstick to My Mastectomy, by Geralyn Lucas (St. Martin's Griffin, 2004). And your best dress: because you're a woman!

The Wisdom of Menopause: Creating Physical and Emotional Health and Healing During the Change, by Christiane Northrup (Bantam, 2006). Whether a river guide or a guide to the next landscape in life, it's good to have someone you trust.

The Year of Magical Thinking, by Joan Didion (Knopf, 2005). The profoundness of a couple, and a family.

The Conversation Continues

The best part of working on this book was the privilege of talking with women around the country who were generous and candid about their story of transfiguration and how it impacted their closets. I cannot begin to express my gratitude to each of them for being a part of this book.

Some women were shy about having their names included and preferred an alias, while others were more comfortable: Peggy Abrams, Paullette Allen, Ruth Ansel, Betsy Ashton, Susan J. Banta, Andy Barnet, Martie Beard, Bev Bennett, Donna Benton, Marilyn Bethany, Sheelah Black, Ali Bogner, Ruth Bolzenius, Aimee Brown, Teresa Canino, Susan Nappa Cocke, Carmen Dell'Orifice, Janis Donnaud, Leah Feldon, Sara Fiedelholz, Karen Fitzgerald, Kathy Ellis Funston, Karen Galland, Lise Gescheidt, Lillian Gilden, Elaine Griffin, Laurie Gross, Terry Grimming, Suzette Hagen, Susan Hall, Dayle Haddon, Scott and Susan Hodin Herlands, Kathie Hightower, Tessa Hooper, Susan Horowitz, Jacqui Jarnes, Jill Johnson, Judy T. Johnson, Kathryn Livingston, Doris Lozada, Marylyn Luna, Beatriz Mallory, Goldie McCray, Roni McGowan, Sallie Mars, Marcia Mentor, Mary Louise Norton, Marilyn Novak-Earley, Debreen Conklin Oliva, Sally Paridis, Didi Pile, Holly Scherer, Lynne D. Schwabe, C.R. Stebbins, Valerie Taloni, Michele Tamtom, Karen Thomas, Penny Tietjen, Carolyn Thompson, Cary Walhof, Julia Ward, Haralee Weintraub, Brenda Willis.

And thanks to designers Nina McLemore, Kay Unger, and Diane von Furstenberg for sharing their style expertise; and to Jenny Cloke, colorist, and Edita Evon and Neil Grupp, stylists at Warren-Tricomi Salon in Greenwich, Connecticut, for sharing their knowledge of hair care; and to Dr. Linda Franks, MD, dermatologist, New York City.

And the conversation continues, as do our lives—and, of course, our closets.

The dogs may bark, but the caravan moves on. —Arab proverb

Bev Bennett started her career in the food department at the *Chicago Sun-Times* where she was active in the Newspaper Guild fight to allow women to remain on the job during pregnancy (Can you imagine?). When she left her job as food editor to be a freelance food writer about a decade ago, she was fighting for better family leave policies. She sees the current period of her life as a blank canvas to fill with work, family, pleasurable activities, and community pursuits.

Marilyn Bethany has since returned from Peru to Upstate New York, where she has cofounded Rural Intelligence.com, a regional culture-and-style news site. Despite working fifteen hours a day at a computer, she has maintained her weight loss by continuing a low-carb regime.

Sheelah Black's interior design firm is thriving "partly because my aged wisdom helps me hear what my clients want and not what I want for them. A silver lining!" (www.sheelahbinc.com)

Carmen Dell'Orifice and Lillian Gilden are casualties of the Bernie Madoff scandal, but carry on despite horrific losses. Carmen has been a model with the Ford Model Agency for sixty-two years and is still going strong. See her on YouTube. Lillian works her independent marketing and branding magic for Wynton Marsalis and other clients at ***connections.

Leah Feldon, former TV host, fashion stylist, journalist, and author, has happily resettled in San Miguel de Allende, Mexico, where she's doing photography that is exhibited in local galleries, building houses, working on a screenplay, and after a recent divorce, has found love again. "So far this is the best chapter of my life . . . I pinch myself every day to make sure I'm not dreaming." (www.leahfeldon.com)

Elaine Griffin, interior designer, became a first-time bride, and also an author with her first book *Design Rules: The Insider's Guide to Becoming Your Own Decorator.*

Susan Hall has built a breathtaking studio on the grounds of the home where she grew up; has married; continues to exhibit her art (Prince Charles and Camilla Parker-Bowles attended a recent show), and has written a creative memoir. Visit her website at www.susanhallart.com.

Kathie Hightower and **Holly Scherer** are international speakers and coauthors of *Help! I'm a Military Spouse—I Get a Life Too!* (2nd edition). Kathie lives on the Oregon coast and Holly is in Washington, D.C. To learn more about their work, visit www.militaryspousehelp.com.

Tessa Hooper is selling the home she has lived in for twenty-three years, where she raised her three children with her now deceased husband, Phil. She is dejunking those closets to start new closets for the rest of her life. They will mostly be packed in a suitcase when she travels the world as a community volunteer. First stop: an orphanage in Tanzania.

Susan Horowitz got a master of fine arts at fifty and is an artist and curator in Los Angeles and New York City. Basic black remains her uniform. (www.susanhorowitz-laprojects.com)

Doris Lozada moved to the United States from Peru as a young woman and started LD Home Remodeling Contractors, Inc., while raising four children on her own. Now that they're grown she's having more fun dressing in color and wearing decorative jewelry. The company thrives, as does she. (www.ld-nyc.com)

Beatriz Mallory and her husband, Gerry, adopted a dog they named Nuit, and had him certified as a therapy dog. Beatriz and Nuit volunteer in hospices. "Bringing life to the days of those with few days of life," Beatriz says, "I'm so proud of my little boy!"

Mary Louise Norton was the fashion director of *Town & Country* for twenty-one years, before she moved to Maine, started an interior design firm called Windemere Studios, and became a widow. Now she is remarried and devotes more time to her life's passion as a painter. (www.mlnortonart.com)

Debreen Oliva utilized her professional organizing skills by teaming up with a fashion image consultant and starting "Don't shop . . . Swap!" clothing parties. She provides closet organization advice prior to the party, and her partner offers style advice to guests during the party. (www.doorganize.com)

Lynne D. Schwabe was owner of Schwabe-May of Charleston, West Virginia, ran her own marketing consulting firm, and is a nationally recognized motivational speaker. She is now the director of development for the National Youth Science Foundation, she does career outplacement counseling for Career Management International, and she is a consultant on a new hedge fund project.

Julia Ward—art consultant, collector, and museum benefactor—and her husband bought a ranch where they built a beautiful home to showcase their art collection. She is now free to pursue her love of fly-fishing, enjoy the changing seasons on the ranch, and return to gardening in her large vegetable and flower garden.

Brenda Willis lost 148 pounds and has kept it off for six years and counting, thanks to daily walks on the treadmill her husband placed in the kitchen. She has turned fifty, been featured on television shows and in magazines (including the *Today* show and *Allure*) for her accomplishment. "I am such a happy girl! Losing the weight has changed my life tremendously! I am healthy, I have energy, and am most positive, even when negative events occur. And I now enjoy shopping for clothes and putting outfits together!" She now hosts weight loss seminars and is writing a book about her life's journey.

For those complaining that no one is making clothes for us gals, check out these companies:

Susan Nappa Cocke was a successful cosmetic executive who married in her early forties and decided she wanted to share more of her life with her husband. She took her design and entrepreneurial talents and created www.proverbialknits .com, which specializes in striking wraps and jewelry for us ladies.

Nina McLemore designs colorful, elegant, separates made for us gals. (www.ninamclemore.com)

Kay Unger creates fun, flirty, sexy, happy (much like her personality) dresses that flatter a woman's body. (www.kayunger.com)

Diane von Furstenberg, in addition to designing womenswear (and, thankfully, continuing to make the wrap dress), is the president of the Council of Fashion Designers of America. (www.dvf.com)

Haralee Weintraub was forty-nine when she experienced instant menopause as a result of chemotherapy. To deal with the hot flashes, she created Haralee, the sleepwear company that makes "Cool Garments for Hot Women." (www.haralee.com)

To join in the conversation on how you want to dress for the rest of your life and to share your own closet stories, visit me online at www.KimJohnsonGross.com, and on Facebook and Twitter, or e-mail me at kim.what2wear@me.com.

Acknowledgments

A special thanks to *More Magazine,* whose mission is to let us gals know how beautiful, cool, stylish, and okay we are as we navigate this next part of our lives, and where I shared my closet stories and those of other women in my "What to Wear for the Rest of Your Life" column. With their permission, I have included a few interviews and expanded versions of stories previously published, most notably "My Bikini and Me" (July, August 2005) in Chapter 1, "Dressing for What's Next" (March 2006) in Chapter 10, and "The Midlife Bride" (June 2007) in Chapter 24.

I am enormously grateful to my publishing team. I'm thrilled that Janis Donnaud, my savvy agent, helped this book find its home with my graceful and wise editor Karen Murgolo and the talented team at Springboard Press/Grand Central Publishing, including Matthew Ballast, Tareth Mitch, Anna Balasi, Laura Jorstad, and Philippa White—and particular thanks for the enthusiasm and support of Jamie Raab, who also published me at Warner Books.

Wayne Wolf continues to bring his design intelligence to my words (www.bluecupcreative.com). Alanna Cavanaugh's lively illustrations jazz up the book and frame the how-did-he-make-me-look-so-good photo, taken by the extraordinary George Lange, that appears on the jacket (www.alannacavannagh.com; www.langephoto.com). Amy Redei artfully illustrates Closet Classics (www.amyredeiillustration.com).

With much love to my sisters Jill Johnson and Susan J. Banta, and Susan's beloved family—Philip, Adriana, Gabrielle, Max, and Sophia—who have all enriched my life.

A big thank-you to David Gross for being a wonderful father to our daughters.

To my friends for your humor, patience, love, and encouragement as I travel through the great divide: Dita Amory, Ruth Ansel, Betsy Ashton, Marilyn Bethany, Ali Bogner, Aimee Brown, Gail and Caesar Bryan, Bob Cooper, Rick Feldman, Susan Horowitz and Sascha Feldman, Debbie Fox, Karen Galland (and Roger), Tony Gantner, Lise Gescheidt and Russ Sollitto, Lillian Gilden, Susan Hall, Mary Louise Hamill, Susan Harrington (and Ted), Tessa Hooper, George and Stephie Lange, Marylyn Luna and Mike Blackaller, Goldie McCray, Becky McDermott (and Tom), Sean McSorley (and team), Dita Naylor-Leyland, Nicholas

Naylor-Leyland, and Teal Mittelstadt, Judith Newman, Sally and Steve, Jesse, Hannah, and Daniel Paridis, Didi Pile, Clifford Ross, Raquel Scott, Winston and Carleen Simone, Cynthia Stebbins, Charlie and Beth Wagner, Jim Winters, my book club in New York City, and the girls in Westport—for starters!

Also, in memory of Peggy Boegner, Kazuko, Agnes Risom, Jerome de Bouyer, Phil Hooper, and Alana DuPont.

And thanks to those who helped me earn a living: Peggy Northrop, Lois Johnson, Joanna Coles, and Marcia Mentor, who brought me into *More Magazine* and encouraged me to write this book.

Jeff Stone, Chic Simple, who remains very chic and very simple.

Caryn Karmatz-Rudy, Grand Central Publishing (formerly Warner Books), who artfully balances the important things in life—a true Life Mentor to many women.

Sonny Mehta, Shelley Wanger, Tony Chirico, Jane Friedman, Pat Johnson, and Paul Bogaards, Knopf—for recognizing Chic Simple as part of the zeitgeist of the 1990s. And it's so 2010—thank you!

Martha Nelson, founder of *InStyle* magazine—a visionary! Thank you for the ride.

Lee Eisenberg and Randy Jones, my bosses at *Esquire*. You always made me feel like a girl, but with something to say!

Lillian Gilden at *** connection, who has connected me professionally with magazines and television opportunities throughout my career.

Judy and Peter Price, *Avenue*—they're legend. It was a unique education in the early days with Michael Shnayerson, Lisa Grunwald, Ray Hooper, Barbara Lish, and Lee Gardiner.

Peter Rogers, Peter Rogers Associates (read the book).

Mary Louise Norton, *Town & Country*—my first Style Mentor, besides my mom.

University of Pennsylvania—my undergraduate years there opened my mind and my world.

Eileen Ford, Ford Model Agency, who put me in front of the camera, but was also proud of me when I decided to move to the other side of the lens.

Illustration Credits

Alanna Cavanagh illustrated the part opening pages, as well as pages 4, 25, 41, 48, 50, 53, 59, 60, 64, 70, 80, 83, 87, 116, 153, 178, 180, 234 and 255.

Amy Redei illustrated pages 2, 8, 30, 33, 68, 75, 90, 95, 96, 100, 105, 107, 109, 113, 119, 123, 127, 128, 130, 138, 140, 147, 150, 159, 175, 177, 183, 197, 198, 208, 212, 214, 217, 220, 231.

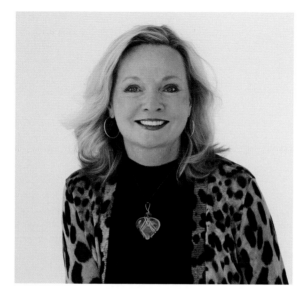

About the Author

Kim Johnson Gross, co-creator of the twenty-five international best-selling *Chic Simple* titles, has been a fashion expert for over thirty years. A former Ford model, fashion editor at *Town & Country* and *Esquire,* and speaker to retail and corporate clients worldwide, she's had her own column in *More* and *InStyle,* and has appeared on national programs, including the *Today* show, CNN, and the *CBS Early Show.* She divides her closets between a home outside of New York City and another in the Rockies.